WEEK BY WEEK PREGNANCY GUIDE FOR MODERN MOMS:

HELPFUL FACTS AND EXPERT TIPS FOR EVERY STAGE OF YOUR JOURNEY

By Naomi Knight

CONTENTS

YOUR FREE GIFT

As a way of saying thanks for your purchase, I'm so happy to offer you the ebook, Pregnancy & Parenting Essentials for FREE.

To get instant access just go to:

https://modernmomspublishing.com/freegift

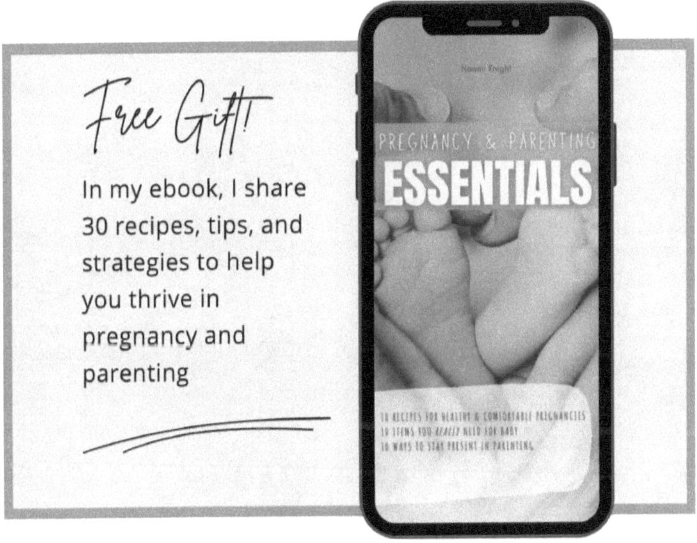

Inside the book, you will discover:

- 10 recipes for healthy and comfortable pregnancies
- 10 items you *really* need for baby
- 10 ways to stay present in parenting

If you want to have my favorite tips on hand during your pregnancy, make sure to grab the free book!

INTRODUCTION: WELCOME TO THE ADVENTURE OF A LIFETIME

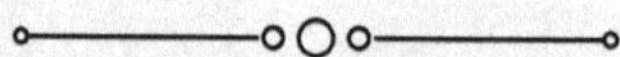

WEEK BY WEEK PREGNANCY GUIDE FOR MODERN MOMS:
HELPFUL FACTS AND EXPERT TIPS FOR EVERY STAGE OF YOUR JOURNEY

By Naomi Knight

Pregnancy is such an extraordinary journey, filled with moments of wonder, excitement, and of course challenges. Whether you're thrilled, nervous, or a bit of both, this guide is here to walk with you every step of the way. We'll explore your pregnancy week by week, offering expert advice, fun tips, and heartfelt encouragement to help you navigate this amazing time in your life.

If you want a book to lay out the basics of pregnancy in an organized and easy to follow way, you found it!

In this guide, you'll find practical information about your baby's development, what changes to expect in your body, and how to prepare for each stage. We'll also include stories from other moms, tips for making pregnancy more enjoyable, and insights to help you feel confident and empowered. Let's embark on this joyful adventure together!

If you're looking for a Pregnancy or First Time Pregnancy book that tells you all the things they *don't* tell you about pregnancy and childbirth then I highly recommend another book I wrote, <u>First Time Pregnancy for Modern Moms: From Planning to Delivery</u>. I'm really proud of how that book teaches moms to make informed decisions, decide on what they want for their birth, and how to advocate for it. So make sure to check that one out if it's of interest!

FIRST TRIMESTER (WEEKS 1-13)

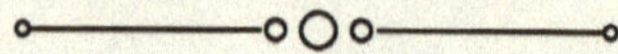

WEEK BY WEEK PREGNANCY GUIDE FOR MODERN MOMS:
HELPFUL FACTS AND EXPERT TIPS FOR EVERY STAGE OF YOUR JOURNEY

By Naomi Knight

WEEKS 1-4: THE ADVENTURE BEGINS!

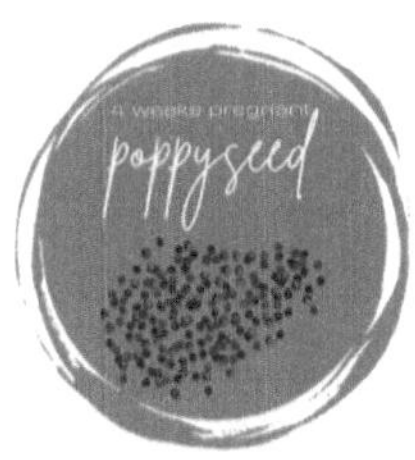

Baby's Size: A teeny-tiny poppy seed

Mother's Symptoms: Fatigue, mild cramping, spotting

What to Expect:

The first few weeks of pregnancy are a **SUCH** whirlwind of emotions and physical changes. You might not even know you're pregnant yet, but your body is already hard at work creating the perfect environment for your baby. During these early days, the fertilized egg implants itself into your uterus, and the journey begins.

If you just found out, CONGRATULATIONS!! 🎉 🍼

Your baby is currently the size of a tiiiiny little poppy seed, but despite its size, it's undergoing incredible changes. Cells are rapidly dividing and forming the foundations for your baby's organs and systems. Hormones like progesterone and hCG are starting to rise, which may cause some early pregnancy symptoms.

Symptoms You Might Experience This Week:

- **Fatigue**: Fatigue is one of the first symptoms many women notice. Your body is expending a lot of energy to support your baby's development, so it's completely normal to feel more tired than usual. It's important to listen to your body and rest whenever you need to. Seriously - snooze it up when you feel drowsy!

- **Mild Cramping and Spotting**: Some women experience mild cramping and light spotting as the embryo implants into the uterus. Don't freak out! This can be concerning, but it's often just a normal part of early pregnancy. However, if you have any concerns, it's always a good idea to check with your healthcare provider.

Preparation Tips:

- **Schedule your first prenatal appointment**: As soon as you suspect you're pregnant, call your healthcare provider to schedule your first prenatal visit. This is an exciting time when you'll discuss your medical history, get a physical exam, and receive your estimated due date.

- **Start prenatal vitamins**: If you haven't started already, now is the time to begin taking a prenatal vitamin with folic acid. Folic acid is crucial in the early weeks for your baby's neural tube development, which will later become the brain and spinal cord. Also, side benefit: get ready for the thickest hair and best nails of your life in this chapter!

- **Healthy Eating**: Consider your diet from the start. A balanced diet rich in fruits, vegetables, whole grains, and lean proteins will help support your baby's growth and your health. Remember, you don't need to eat for two just yet, but focusing on nutrient-rich foods is key.

Personal Story:

Many moms describe finding out they're pregnant as a surreal moment. For some, it's a sudden realization—missing a period and a quick test confirming what they hoped (or suspected). Others recount a more gradual awareness as symptoms like fatigue and queasiness set in. Emma, a first-time mom, shared, "I just knew something was different. I took a test the day after my missed period and, when I saw those two lines, I burst into tears of joy. It was the start of something incredible." For me, it was the faintest line after a missed period. I will never forget the way it instantly shifted my perspective and thinking from "we are trying to do this" to "we are doing this!" From "I'd like to be a mom" to "I'm going to be a mom." It felt like being thrown onto a super fun roller coaster and I'm still on the ride!

WEEK 5: THE HEARTBEAT BEGINS

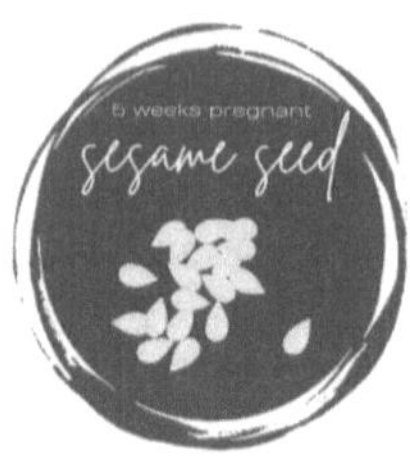

Baby's Size: A sesame seed

Mother's Symptoms: Fatigue, slight nausea, heightened sense of smell

What to Expect:

At week 5, your baby is still incredibly small—just the size of a sesame seed—but **big** changes are happening! This is the week when the heart begins to form and beat, marking a major milestone in your baby's development. The neural tube, which will become the brain and spinal cord, is also starting to close, laying the foundation for your baby's nervous system.

For you, the early signs of pregnancy may be kicking in. If you didn't yet last week, you might start feeling more tired than usual as your body works hard to support your growing baby. A heightened sense of smell is common, and certain odors might start to bother you.

More on the Symptoms You Might Experience This Week:

- **Fatigue**: The fatigue is gonna be real for a while. You may feel more tired than usual, and that's because your body is working overtime to support your baby's rapid development. Listen to your body and rest when you need to. Seriously, nap it up, girl!

- **Slight Nausea**: Nausea might start to make an appearance, though it's still early. Eating small, frequent meals and avoiding strong smells can help. Also, make sure you eat right away in the morning. The nausea likes to rear its ugly head when you're super hungry. Which is so counter-intuitive. Right when you want to eat, you feel so nauseous that the thought of food makes you want to barf!

- **Heightened Sense of Smell**: Your sense of smell may become more acute, and you might find that certain odors are suddenly off-putting. This can be very intense but it is a normal part of early pregnancy.

Preparation Tips:

- **Schedule your first prenatal visit**: If you haven't already, now is the time to schedule your first prenatal appointment, usually around 8 weeks. This will give you a chance to check in with your healthcare provider and confirm your pregnancy.

- **Start taking prenatal vitamins**: If you haven't started yet, make sure to begin taking a prenatal vitamin with folic acid to support your baby's development.
- **Rest**: I know I keep saying this:) And you'll hear it plenty more throughout the book! Fatigue is common at this stage, so make sure you're getting enough rest. Take naps if you need to, and don't be afraid to go to bed earlier than usual. It feels so good to give your body sleep when it asks for it, so really try to listen to your body and, if you can lay down for a 15 minute nap even, that's great.

WEEK 6: RAPID GROWTH AND MORNING SICKNESS

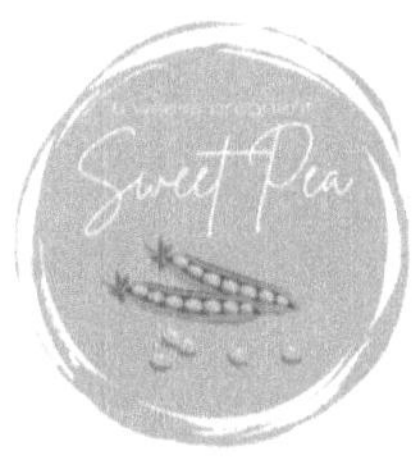

Baby's Size: A sweet little pea

Mother's Symptoms: Morning sickness, breast tenderness, fatigue

What to Expect:

By week 6, your baby is growing rapidly and has doubled in size, now about the size of a sweet pea. This is a busy week for development—your baby's heart is beating around 100 to 160 times per minute, and the major organs, such as the lungs and liver, are beginning to take shape. Tiny buds are forming where the arms and legs will be, and the neural tube continues to develop.

This is also when many women start to experience more pronounced symptoms. Morning sickness might kick into high gear, and you could feel queasy throughout the day. Your breasts may feel tender and swollen as they prepare for breastfeeding, and fatigue may still be a constant companion.

More on the Symptoms You Might Experience This Week:

- **Morning Sickness**: If you're gonna get morning sickness at all (a lot of women don't and that's totally okay) you will probably be feeling it by now. Morning sickness is common around this time and can vary from mild nausea to more intense queasiness. Try to eat small, frequent meals and stay hydrated. Ginger tea, crackers, and peppermint can be helpful.

- **Breast Tenderness**: Your breasts are preparing for their role in feeding your baby, so tenderness and swelling are normal. Wearing a supportive bra can help ease discomfort. I cannot tell you how many women I know figured out they were pregnant because someone said their chi-chis were looking especially…large, lol. My sister, for example, hadn't noticed her period passed. She went out with some girlfriends and they all were like, 'dang girl!''. My sister thought a little more about it and decided to drink soda water that night. Sure enough, she was 6 weeks pregnant with my nephew!

- **Fatigue**: Your body is still adjusting to the demands of pregnancy, so continue to prioritize rest.

Preparation Tips:

- **Plan your pregnancy announcement**: You might start thinking about how and when you want to announce your pregnancy to family and friends. Some women choose to wait until the end of the first trimester, **but it's entirely up to you.** If you want my personal opinion, I would have some fun with this if I was under 35. Over 35, and it's definitely best to wait until you're in the clear (as in passed 12 weeks). Miscarriages are way common over 35, ya'll! They're hard to get through but they'd be way easier if we talked about them and normalized them more.

- **Stock up on snacks**: Having healthy snacks on hand can help manage morning sickness and keep your energy levels up. Nuts, fruits, and whole-grain crackers are great options.

- **Research prenatal exercise**: Staying active during pregnancy is beneficial for both you and your baby. Look into prenatal yoga, walking, or swimming as low-impact options to keep you fit and healthy. If you already have an exercise regimen, you can most likely exercise as long as you want to in your pregnancy, as long as you are comfortable and your doctor says it's okay. I taught 1 hour group exercise classes until 8 ½ months.

WEEK 7: TAKING SHAPE

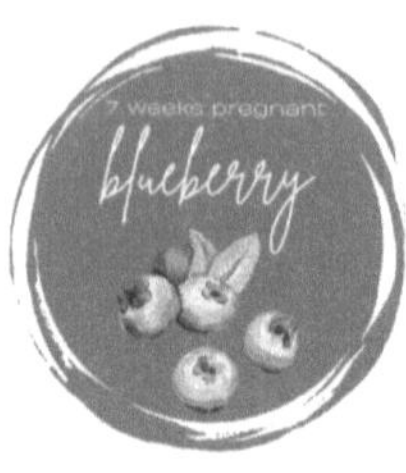

Baby's Size: A tiny blueberry

Mother's Symptoms: Increased nausea, food aversions, mood swings

What to Expect:

Your baby is now about the size of a blueberry, and even though they're still tiny, they're growing fast! The brain is developing rapidly, with new cells forming at an astonishing rate. Your baby's face is starting to take shape, with the beginnings of eyes, nostrils, and ears. The arms and legs are starting to lengthen, and small hands and feet are forming, though they look more like paddles at this stage.

For many women, week 7 is when pregnancy symptoms really start to intensify. Nausea might be more persistent, and you may develop strong food aversions. Mood swings are also common as your hormones fluctuate, making you feel like you're on an emotional rollercoaster.

More on the Symptoms You Might Experience This Week:

- **Increased Nausea**: Morning sickness might be more noticeable now, and certain foods or smells might trigger it. Eating bland foods like toast or plain rice can help, as can ginger and peppermint. My girlfriends who had kids before me advised me to keep something to get in my belly as soon as I woke up, by the bed. That worked for me - as long as I had some soda crackers upon waking, I'd be okay. But if I got too hungry too quick, it was over and I'd be hurling for the next half hour - MISERABLE! Find what works for you (crackers, cereal bar) and keep it on the nightstand.

- **Food Aversions**: You might find that foods you once loved are now unappealing - and in some cases, full on appalling - while you crave things you never cared for before. Go with your cravings when possible, and don't worry if your diet isn't perfect right now—just do your best to eat what you can. A lot of women actually lose weight in this period because of the morning sickness and food aversions, so just do your best and eat when it works!

- **Mood Swings**: Hormonal changes can cause mood swings that leave you feeling up and down. Remember, it's normal to feel emotional, and it's okay to reach out for support if you need it. I found laughing it off worked best! I'd notice how emotional I was and then I'd take a moment to just let myself be tickled at a what a sap I was from all the hormones.

Preparation Tips:

- **Experiment with foods**: If food aversions are making it hard to eat, try experimenting with different foods to see what works for you. Sometimes, cold foods are easier to tolerate, or you might find comfort in simple, bland meals.
- **Stay hydrated**: Drinking plenty of water is crucial, especially if you're dealing with nausea and vomiting. Sipping water throughout the day can help, and if plain water isn't appealing, try adding a splash of juice or a slice of lemon. This wasn't hard for me because I found myself much thirstier. It was easier to drink more water - I craved it!
- **Plan for the weeks ahead**: As your pregnancy progresses, start thinking about your prenatal care and any upcoming appointments. Make sure you're comfortable with your healthcare provider and that you have a good support system in place!

WEEK 8: MOVING TOWARD THE FETUS STAGE

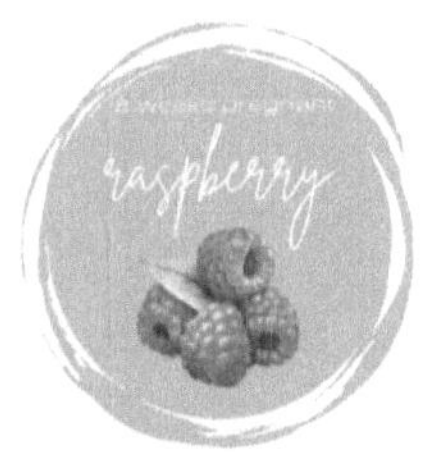

Baby's Size: A plump raspberry

Mother's Symptoms: Bloating, frequent urination, heightened emotions

What to Expect:

By week 8, your baby has grown to about the size of a raspberry and is almost ready to transition from embryo to fetus. All of their major organs and body systems are in place, and they're continuing to grow and develop rapidly. The tail that was present during the earlier weeks is disappearing, and your baby is starting to look more human every day. Momma, you are building a tiny human in there!!

You might notice that your clothes are starting to feel a bit tighter as your uterus expands, though it's still early for most women to start showing. Bloating and frequent urination are common symptoms as your body adjusts to the increasing demands of pregnancy. Your emotions might be running high as well, with mood swings continuing to be a regular part of your day. Allow yourself some grace here!

More on the Symptoms You Might Experience This Week:

- **Bloating**: Bloating is common as your body retains more fluids and your digestive system slows down due to the hormone progesterone. Wearing loose, comfortable clothing can help, and try to eat small, frequent meals to ease digestion.
- **Frequent Urination**: As your uterus grows, it puts pressure on your bladder, causing you to need to pee more often. It's important to stay hydrated, but you might want to limit fluids before bedtime to reduce nighttime trips to the bathroom.
- **Heightened Emotions**: Pregnancy hormones can cause your emotions to fluctuate, and you might find yourself crying at commercials or feeling overwhelmed by small things. Remember, it's all part of the journey, and it's okay to feel whatever you're feeling.

Preparation Tips:

- **Start a pregnancy journal** Now that your pregnancy is well underway, consider starting a journal to document your experiences, thoughts, and feelings. It's a great way to capture memories and track milestones.

- **Listen to Positive Affirmations for Pregnancy & Labor:** This immensely helped my nerves and anxiety during the emotional times. When my brain was in overdrive and I couldn't quite calm it, positive affirmations helped bring me back down to the here and now so I could enjoy my pregnancy. It also really helped me feel a bond with my baby. That comes later when you start showing and definitely after you feel the first kick. But I found, listening to affirmations helped me bond with my baby much earlier.

- **Think about maternity clothes:** If you're starting to feel bloated or uncomfortable in your regular clothes, it might be time to start thinking about maternity wear. Look for pieces that are stretchy, comfortable, and can grow with you.

- **Connect with other moms:** Joining a pregnancy group, either online or in person, can be a great way to connect with other moms-to-be. Sharing experiences, advice, and support can make the journey even more special.

Personal Story:

Jennifer, who was pregnant with her second child, shared how she dealt with bloating and frequent urination: "Around week 8, I really started to notice the bloating—it felt like I was already showing, even though it was just bloating. I also couldn't believe how often I needed to use the bathroom! I started wearing looser clothes and making sure I stayed hydrated, especially during the day so I wouldn't have to get up too much at night. It was a relief to know these symptoms were normal, and I just took it one day at a time."

WEEK 9: TINY LIMBS AND BIG CHANGES

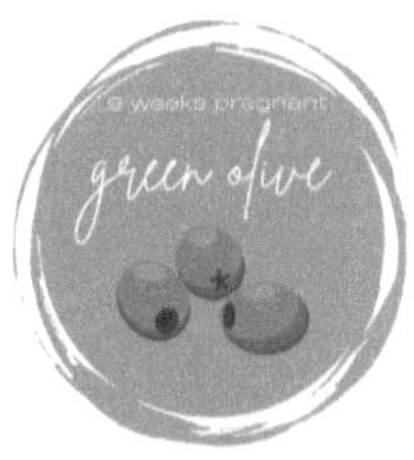

Baby's Size: A green olive

Mother's Symptoms: Bloating, fatigue, stronger food aversions

What to Expect:

At week 9, your baby is about the size of a green olive and is officially considered a fetus. The most critical stages of development are now behind you, and your baby's organs are fully formed and beginning to function. Tiny fingers and toes are starting to appear, and your baby's facial features are becoming more distinct, with the formation of the nose, mouth, and eyes.

You might still be feeling the effects of early pregnancy, with symptoms like bloating and fatigue persisting. Food aversions could be stronger than ever, making it hard to enjoy meals you used to love. These symptoms are all part of your body's way of adjusting to the rapid changes happening inside you. You are getting close to the end of these symptoms being so intense so hang in there! In about three weeks, things will shift and get more comfortable.

More on the Symptoms You Might Experience This Week:

- **Bloating**: Bloating is common as your digestive system slows down due to increased progesterone. Wearing loose, comfortable clothing can help, and drinking plenty of water can ease bloating.
- **Fatigue**: Your body is still working hard to support your baby's growth, so don't be surprised if you feel more tired than usual. Rest whenever you can, and don't hesitate to take it easy.
- **Food Aversions**: Strong food aversions might make it challenging to eat certain foods. It's okay to avoid them for now and focus on what you can tolerate. Sometimes, simple, bland foods like crackers or toast can be easier to handle.

Preparation Tips:

- **Research prenatal vitamins**: Ensure that your prenatal vitamin includes all the essential nutrients like folic acid, iron, and DHA. These are crucial for your baby's development, especially in the early stages.
- **Plan meals around your aversions**: If you're struggling with food aversions, try planning meals

around what you can tolerate. Sometimes, cold foods or mild flavors are more manageable. Don't worry if your diet isn't perfect—just focus on getting through this phase.

- **Stay connected with your healthcare provider**: Regular communication with your healthcare provider is essential. Don't hesitate to reach out if you have concerns about your symptoms or need advice on managing them.

WEEK 10: FROM EMBRYO TO FETUS

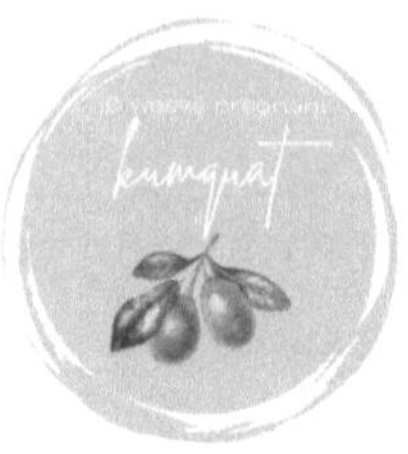

Baby's Size: A juicy kumquat

Mother's Symptoms: Frequent urination, heightened sense of smell, emotional swings

What to Expect:

By week 10, your baby is the size of a kumquat and is growing quickly. The vital organs, including the liver, kidneys, intestines, and brain, are all functioning. Bones and cartilage are forming, and tiny nails are starting to grow on the fingers and toes. Your baby is even practicing swallowing!

As your uterus continues to expand, you may find yourself needing to use the bathroom more frequently. Your heightened sense of smell might make certain odors unbearable, and you might experience emotional swings due to the ongoing hormonal shifts. It's a time of big changes, both for your baby and for you.

More on the Symptoms You Might Experience This Week:

- **Frequent Urination**: As your uterus grows, it puts pressure on your bladder, causing more frequent bathroom trips. Stay hydrated, but try to limit fluids in the evening to reduce nighttime trips.

- **Heightened Sense of Smell**: This can be a blessing and a curse. While you might enjoy certain scents more, others might become intolerable. Avoid strong smells that bother you and try to keep your environment as pleasant as possible.

- **Emotional Swings**: Hormones can cause your emotions to fluctuate. One minute you might feel elated, and the next, you're in tears. These emotional swings are normal, so give yourself grace and reach out for support if needed.

Preparation Tips:

- **First trimester screening**: Around this time, your healthcare provider may offer screening tests to check for chromosomal abnormalities. These tests are optional, so discuss your options with your provider to determine what's best for you.

- **Prepare for maternity wear**: If your regular clothes are starting to feel tight, it might be time to invest in some maternity wear. Comfort is key, and there are plenty of stylish options available to keep you feeling good as your body changes. Don't forget, people only wear maternity clothes for a few months so hand-me-downs are usually still in great shape! If you have friends that got pregnant before you, they probably have a box for you. If not, check out the second hand and consignment stores for deals. There is nothing wrong with buying maternity clothes new either! But if money's tight, a mix of both used and new clothes or even all used clothes will totally work.

- **Practice self-care**: This is a great time to focus on self-care. Whether it's a warm bath, a relaxing walk, or just some quiet time with a book, take time to nurture yourself during this period of rapid change.

WEEK 11: GROWTH AND REFINEMENT

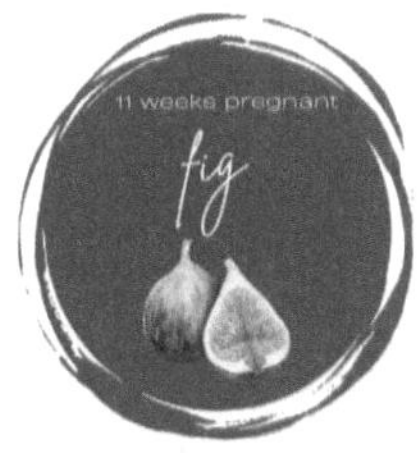

Baby's Size: A fig

Mother's Symptoms: Less nausea, increased appetite, mild cramping

What to Expect:

At week 11, your baby is the size of a fig and continues to grow rapidly. The bones in their face are forming, and the ears are moving into their final position. Your baby's head still makes up about half of their total length, but the body is catching up. They're also starting to develop more distinct fingers and toes, and the hair follicles, tooth buds, and nail beds are beginning to form.

You might start to notice a decrease in nausea as you approach the end of the first trimester. However, mild cramping is common as your uterus continues to expand. Your appetite might also begin to increase as your body demands more energy to support your baby's growth.

More on the Symptoms You Might Experience This Week:

- **Less Nausea**: Hopefully, as the placenta takes over hormone production, you might notice that your nausea is starting to ease. If you're still experiencing morning sickness, it should begin to taper off in the coming weeks. If it's getting you down just remember, if you're gonna get morning sickness at all, it's good to get it BAD, lol. That means your body made a good dose of hormones for your baby development and the chance of miscarriage is way lower.

- **Increased Appetite**: With your nausea subsiding, you might find your appetite returning. Focus on nutrient-rich foods that will fuel both you and your baby. It's okay to indulge in cravings occasionally, but try to maintain a balanced diet.

- **Mild Cramping**: Mild cramping is a normal part of your uterus expanding. It can feel like period cramps and is usually nothing to worry about. However, if the cramping is severe or accompanied by bleeding, contact your healthcare provider.

Preparation Tips:

- **Schedule your next prenatal appointment**: If you haven't already, schedule your next prenatal appointment. This will likely include an ultrasound to check on your baby's growth and development.

- **Update your diet**: As your appetite returns, consider updating your diet to include a variety of fruits, vegetables, whole grains, and lean proteins. This will help ensure you and your baby are getting the nutrients you need. It will also help your energy levels. The heartburn that gets worse as pregnancy progresses will also be much easier to manage if you're eating a cleaner diet. Lastly, it's much easier to recover from your pregnancy if you eat a whole 30 or anti-inflammatory type diet. It's just a win-win-win situation to eat right once your morning sickness clears so I encourage you to try. There's a free gift at the beginning of this book with some great recipes.

- **Start thinking about prenatal classes**: Now is a good time to start researching prenatal classes in your area. Whether it's childbirth education, breastfeeding, or newborn care, these classes can help you feel more prepared for what's ahead.

WEEK 12: ENTERING THE SECOND TRIMESTER

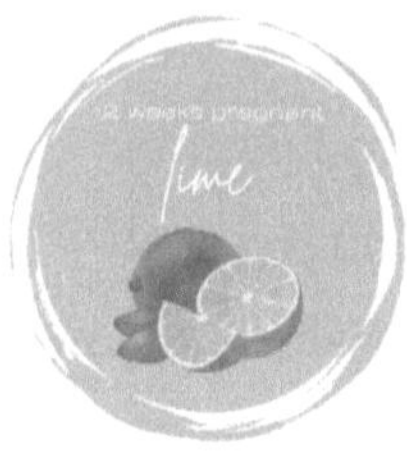

Baby's Size: A lime

Mother's Symptoms: Bloating, occasional headaches, glowing skin

What to Expect:

Congratulations! At week 12, your baby is about the size of a lime and has officially graduated from embryo to fetus. This is a significant milestone as your baby's development continues to accelerate. The digestive system is starting to practice contraction movements, and the bone marrow is producing white blood cells. Your baby is also beginning to develop reflexes, so they might start making spontaneous movements that you can't feel yet.

You might experience some bloating as your uterus continues to grow, and occasional headaches are common due to the increased blood volume in your body. On a positive note, many women begin to notice that their skin looks more radiant, often referred to as the "pregnancy glow."

More on the Symptoms You Might Experience This Week:

- **Bloating**: Man, if I had a dollar for every time I had to tell you about bloating I'd be loaded;) As your uterus expands, it can press on your intestines, leading to bloating. Eating smaller meals and staying hydrated can help alleviate this discomfort.

- **Occasional Headaches**: Hormonal changes and increased blood volume can lead to headaches. Make sure you're drinking enough water, and try to rest in a dark, quiet room if a headache strikes.

- **Glowing Skin**: The pregnancy glow is real! Increased blood circulation gives your skin a rosy hue, and hormonal changes can lead to oilier, more radiant skin. Enjoy this perk of pregnancy and embrace your natural beauty.

Preparation Tips:

- **Prepare for your second trimester**: As you near the end of the first trimester, start preparing for the changes that come with the second trimester. You'll likely have more energy and start to show, so consider updating your wardrobe and planning activities you enjoy.

- **Document your journey**: Now that you're entering a new phase of pregnancy, consider documenting your journey with photos, journal entries, or even a blog. It's a special time, and you'll love looking back on these memories.

- **Review your budget**: If you haven't already, start budgeting for baby expenses. This includes setting aside money for big-ticket items like a crib, stroller, and car seat. It's also a good time to start thinking about saving for maternity leave if applicable.

WEEK 13: WRAPPING UP THE FIRST TRIMESTER

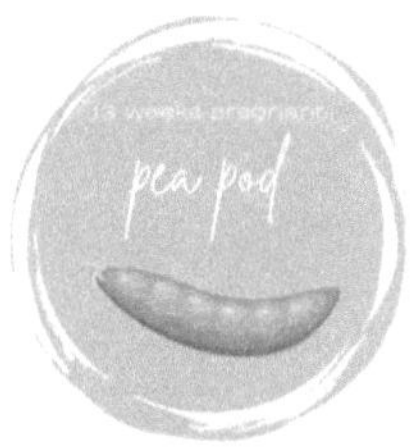

Baby's Size: A pea pod

Mother's Symptoms: Reduced fatigue, renewed energy, slight weight gain

What to Expect:

At week 13, your baby is about the size of a pea pod, and you've reached the final week of your first trimester. Your baby's organs and systems are fully formed and now entering a phase of rapid growth and maturation. The intestines are moving into their final position, and your baby's vocal cords are developing. Your little one is also starting to practice movements like swallowing and sucking.

Hopefully by now, the fatigue and nausea of the first trimester are beginning to lift, replaced by a renewed sense of energy. Slight weight gain is normal as your body continues to support your growing baby. Many women start to feel more like themselves again as they enter the second trimester.

It's totally up to you when you want to tell people you are pregnant. The risk of miscarriage takes a massive dive after this week, so if you have been waiting for that reason, you're in the clear.

More on the Symptoms You Might Experience This Week:

- **Reduced Fatigue:** As you transition into the second trimester, you may find that your energy levels are starting to improve. Take advantage of this time to get things done, but also remember to continue prioritizing rest when needed.

- **Renewed Energy:** With your energy returning, you might feel more motivated to exercise, socialize, and tackle projects. It's a great time to engage in activities you enjoy, whether it's a gentle workout, a hobby, or spending time with loved ones.

- **Slight Weight Gain:** A slight increase in weight is normal at this stage as your baby and uterus grow. Focus on eating balanced meals and listening to your body's hunger cues. Remember, every pregnancy is different, and weight gain varies from person to person.

Preparation Tips:

- **Celebrate the end of the first trimester:** You've made it through the first trimester, and that's something to celebrate! Whether it's a small treat for yourself or a special dinner with your partner, take a moment to acknowledge this milestone.
- **Plan for upcoming appointments:** As you move into the second trimester, you'll have regular prenatal appointments to monitor your baby's growth. Plan ahead for these visits and any tests or screenings that might be offered.
- **Continue prenatal care:** Keep up with your prenatal vitamins, healthy eating, and regular exercise. These habits are important throughout your pregnancy and will help you feel your best as you move forward.

Personal Story:

Emily, who had just completed her first trimester, shared her experience: "Reaching week 13 felt like such an accomplishment. I was finally starting to feel more energetic, and my nausea was almost completely gone. I celebrated by going out to dinner with my husband—my first real meal out in weeks! It was a relief to be entering the second trimester, knowing that my baby was growing strong and healthy."

SECOND TRIMESTER (WEEKS 14-27)

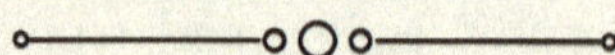

WEEK BY WEEK PREGNANCY GUIDE FOR MODERN MOMS:
HELPFUL FACTS AND EXPERT TIPS FOR EVERY STAGE OF YOUR JOURNEY

By Naomi Knight

WEEK 14: THE HONEYMOON PHASE BEGINS

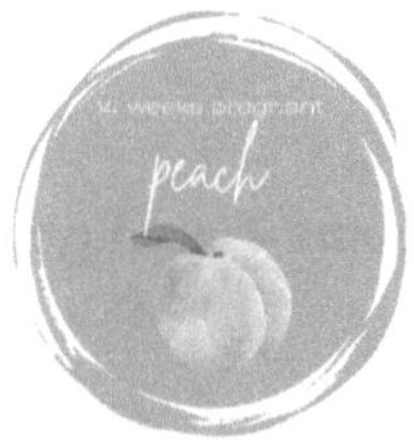

Baby's Size: A peach

Mother's Symptoms: Energy boost, reduced nausea, glowing skin

What to Expect:

Welcome to week 14, the official start of your second trimester! This is often called the "honeymoon phase" of pregnancy because many of the more challenging symptoms from the first trimester, like nausea and fatigue, begin to ease up. Your baby is now about the size of a peach and continues to grow at a rapid pace. Their neck is getting longer, allowing the head to sit more upright, and the arms are starting to grow in proportion to the rest of the body. The liver is producing bile, and the spleen is helping to produce red blood cells.

You may start to feel more like yourself again as your energy levels increase, and you might notice your skin starting to glow—a common effect of increased blood circulation and pregnancy hormones. This is a great time to embrace the positive changes and enjoy this new phase of your pregnancy.

More on the Symptoms You Might Experience This Week:

- **Energy Boost**: With the fatigue of the first trimester behind you, you may find yourself with a renewed sense of energy. Use this time to catch up on things you may have put off, whether it's organizing your home, planning for the baby, or simply enjoying time with loved ones.

- **Reduced Nausea**: For many women, nausea finally subsides around this time, making it easier to enjoy meals and maintain a balanced diet. If your nausea persists, try sticking to small, frequent meals and continue to avoid any known triggers.

- **Glowing Skin**: The so-called "pregnancy glow" is a real thing, and it's due to increased blood flow and hormonal changes. Enjoy the compliments that come your way and take care of your skin with gentle, hydrating products.

Preparation Tips:

- **Schedule a prenatal checkup**: Around this time, you'll likely have a prenatal checkup where your healthcare provider will check your baby's heartbeat and measure your belly. Use this opportunity to ask any questions you have about your pregnancy.

- **Update your wardrobe**: If you haven't already, now might be the time to invest in some maternity clothing. As your belly grows, you'll appreciate comfortable and supportive options that accommodate your changing shape.

- **Start thinking about prenatal exercise**: With your energy levels up, consider starting or continuing a prenatal exercise routine. Activities like walking, swimming, and prenatal yoga can help you stay fit and prepare your body for childbirth.

WEEK 15: TINY MOVEMENTS AND BIG PLANS

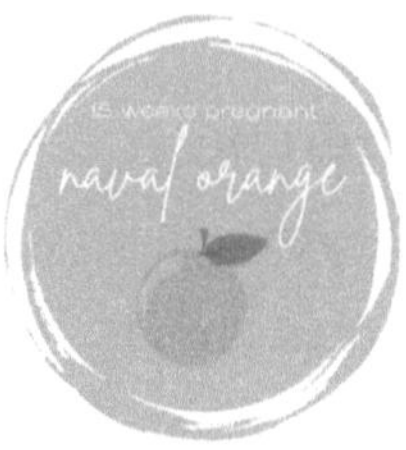

Baby's Size: A navel orange

Mother's Symptoms: Increased appetite, less fatigue, the occasional headache

What to Expect:

By week 15, your baby is about the size of a navel orange and is becoming more active. Their legs are now longer than their arms, and they're starting to move those tiny limbs more frequently. Although you might not feel these movements just yet, they're practicing for the big day when you will. Your baby's skin is still very thin, and blood vessels can be seen beneath the surface. The ears are positioned on the sides of the head, and the eyes are continuing to move closer together.

For you, the second trimester continues to bring more comfort. You may notice an increase in your appetite as your body works hard to nourish your growing baby. While fatigue is generally less of an issue now, occasional headaches can still occur due to hormonal changes and increased blood volume.

More on the Symptoms You Might Experience This Week:

- **Increased Appetite**: As your baby grows, so does your appetite. Focus on nutrient-dense foods that provide the vitamins and minerals both you and your baby need. It's okay to indulge cravings occasionally, but try to maintain a balanced diet overall.

- **Less Fatigue**: Many women find that the overwhelming fatigue of the first trimester is now a thing of the past. Woo-hoo! Use this time to engage in activities you enjoy, whether it's a hobby, spending time outdoors, or connecting with friends.

- **Occasional Headaches**: Hormonal shifts, dehydration, or stress can lead to headaches. Make sure you're drinking enough water and getting plenty of rest. If headaches persist, consult your healthcare provider for safe remedies.

Preparation Tips:

- **Start thinking about your birth plan**: It's not too early to start considering your preferences for labor and delivery. Begin researching different birth options, pain management techniques, and discuss these with your healthcare provider. In the book <u>First Time Pregnancy for Modern Moms</u>, we really dive into these topics so you can make informed decisions for your and your baby's care. I highly recommend checking it out if you're interested in learning all the things they don't tell you in regards to navigating your pregnancy journey through the medical industrial complex.

- **Plan your baby shower**: If you're planning to have a baby shower, now is a great time to start thinking about the details. Whether you're organizing it yourself or leaving it to a friend or family member, it's a fun way to celebrate your pregnancy.

- **Look into childbirth education classes**: Many classes fill up quickly, so consider signing up for a childbirth education course in the coming weeks. These classes can help you feel more prepared for labor and delivery, and give you a chance to ask questions in a supportive environment.

WEEK 16: FEELING THE FIRST FLUTTERS

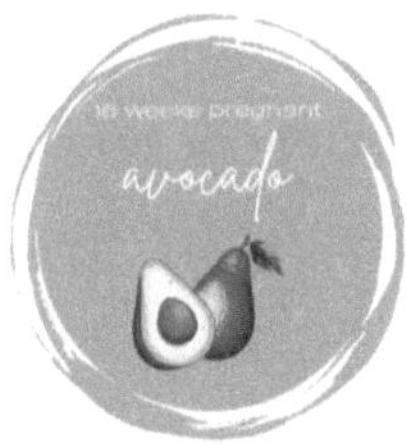

Baby's Size: An avocado

Mother's Symptoms: Feeling baby move, lower back pain, increased blood flow

What to Expect:

At week 16, your baby is about the size of an avocado and is developing rapidly. Their eyes are moving closer to the front of the face, and the ears are almost in their final position. The scalp pattern is beginning to form, although there isn't any hair just yet. Inside, your baby's heart is pumping about 25 quarts of blood each day, and their tiny muscles are strengthening, allowing them to make more purposeful movements.

One of the most exciting developments this week (shoot, in this trimester!) is that you might start to feel your baby move! These first flutters, often described as feeling like bubbles or butterflies in your belly, are known as quickening. Another way to describe it is like the sensation of your eye twitching but in your belly. It's a magical moment that many moms remember for the rest of their lives. You might also start to notice some lower back pain as your belly grows and your center of gravity shifts. Make sure to stretch more and not sit for too long if lower back pain is an issue for you!

More on the Symptoms You Might Experience This Week:

- **Feeling Baby Move**: Those first movements can be subtle, so you might mistake them for gas or muscle twitches. As the weeks go by, these movements will become more pronounced and frequent, offering a constant reminder of the little life growing inside you. It's trippy! When you just sit there and watch your belly move. Enjoy it - there is no other sensation like it and it's over before you know it.

- **Lower Back Pain**: As your baby grows, your posture may change, leading to lower back pain. Consider using a pregnancy pillow for support when sleeping, and practice good posture throughout the day to minimize discomfort.

- **Increased Blood Flow**: Pregnancy increases blood flow to support your growing baby, which can cause your skin to look more flushed and your veins to appear more prominent. This is perfectly normal and a sign that your body is working hard to support your pregnancy.

Preparation Tips:

- **Start a pregnancy journal**: If you haven't already, consider starting a journal to document your thoughts, feelings, and experiences during pregnancy. It's a wonderful way to capture memories and reflect on this special time.
- **Consider a maternity support belt**: If you're experiencing lower back pain, a maternity support belt can help alleviate discomfort by providing extra support to your growing belly and lower back. I found this very helpful later in my third trimester especially.
- **Plan some "me time"**: With your energy levels up and before your baby arrives, take time to indulge in activities that bring you joy. Whether it's a day at the spa, a favorite hobby, or a quiet afternoon with a good book, these moments of self-care are important.

WEEK 17: GROWING STRONG AND LOOKING AHEAD

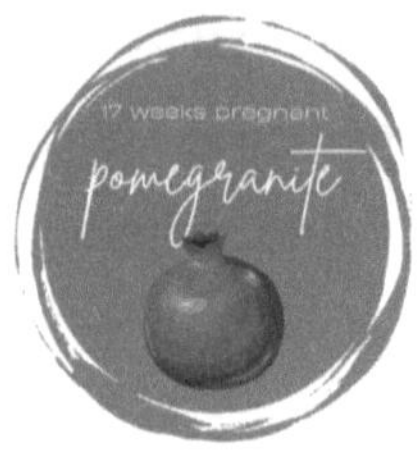

Baby's Size: A pomegranate

Mother's Symptoms: Round ligament pain, visible baby bump, glowing skin

What to Expect:

By week 17, your baby is about the size of a pomegranate and is continuing to grow stronger every day. Their skeleton is changing from soft cartilage to bone, and they're developing a layer of fat beneath the skin, which will help regulate their body temperature after birth. The umbilical cord, which provides your baby with nutrients and oxygen, is getting thicker and stronger.

You might notice that your baby bump is becoming more visible, and your clothes might be feeling a bit snug. This is also when some women start experiencing round ligament pain, a sharp pain or jabbing feeling in the lower belly or groin area that's caused by the stretching of the ligaments that support your uterus. On the bright side, your skin might be glowing, thanks to increased blood circulation and the hormonal changes of pregnancy.

More on the Symptoms You Might Experience This Week:

- **Round Ligament Pain**: This pain is common as your uterus grows and the ligaments stretch to accommodate your baby. It can be uncomfortable but is usually not a cause for concern. Moving slowly and avoiding sudden movements can help minimize discomfort.

- **Visible Baby Bump**: Your belly is likely becoming more pronounced, and you may start to feel like you truly "look" pregnant. Embrace this change and consider taking weekly photos to document your growing bump. I found that once I was showing, things got much more exciting! A baby bump is so cute to wear - there are some fun maternity clothes out there! And this is when it's not just you and a few who know you are pregnant. When you can't hide it, everybody knows and people get excited for you. Once I gained some weight in the first trimester, I just felt frumpy, and that's sure what people saw because I wasn't telling anyone I was expecting. But once the baby bump was there, I felt the opposite of frumpy. I rocked that baby bump, and you should too!

- **Glowing Skin:** The pregnancy glow continues, thanks to the extra blood flow and hormones that keep your skin looking radiant. Keep up your skincare routine, and enjoy the compliments! Between this and the baby bump, you must rock this look!! Enjoy momma. You earned it.

Preparation Tips:

- **Think about baby names**: If you haven't started already, now is a great time to begin discussing baby names. Make a list of your favorites, and consider meanings, family traditions, or simply what sounds best to you and your partner.
- **Start thinking about the nursery**: With your baby bump growing, it's time to start planning the nursery. Think about themes, colors, and furniture you might need. It's an exciting way to prepare for your baby's arrival. Don't let this one scare you if you live in a small space. You can have a baby anywhere! A nursery can be in the corner of your apartment and still be comfortable and look adorable.
- **Connect with your partner**: Take time to connect with your partner and discuss your hopes, concerns, and plans for the future. Whether it's a casual conversation over dinner or a planned date night, nurturing your relationship is important as you prepare to become parents together.

Personal Story:

Katie, who was expecting her first child, shared her experience with round ligament pain: "I remember feeling a sharp pain in my lower belly when I stood up too quickly, and it really scared me at first. But after talking to my doctor, I learned it was just round ligament pain—totally normal as everything stretches to make room for the baby. I started moving more slowly and being more mindful of my posture, which really helped. It's all part of the process, and it was actually kind of comforting to know my body was changing to support my baby."

WEEK 18: HEARING YOUR HEARTBEAT

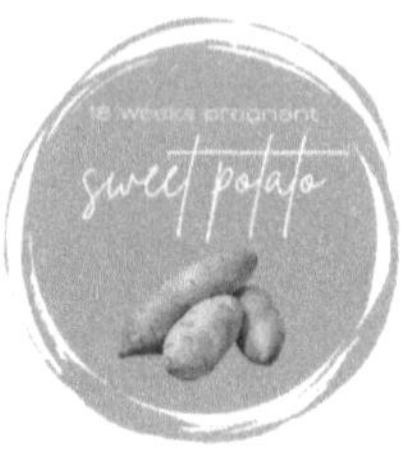

Baby's Size: A sweet potato

Mother's Symptoms: Backaches, round ligament pain, increased appetite

What to Expect:

At week 18, your baby is about the size of a sweet potato and is undergoing significant developments, particularly in their senses. The most exciting news is that your baby's ears are now developed enough to hear sounds from the outside world. This means they can hear your heartbeat, your voice, and even music you play. Their nervous system is maturing, and the myelin, a protective coating around nerves, is starting to form, which will continue to develop for years after birth.

As your baby grows and your belly expands, you might start to experience more noticeable backaches and round ligament pain. Your center of gravity is shifting, which can cause strain on your lower back. Additionally, your increased appetite may become more apparent as your body requires more energy to support your growing baby.

More on the Symptoms You Might Experience This Week:

- **Backaches:** The growing weight of your baby can put pressure on your spine, leading to discomfort. Maintaining good posture and incorporating gentle stretching exercises can help alleviate the strain. Consider using a pregnancy pillow at night to support your back and growing belly.

- **Round Ligament Pain:** As your uterus grows, the ligaments that support it stretch, which can cause sharp pains on one or both sides of your abdomen. Moving slowly when standing up or changing positions can help minimize these pains.

- **Increased Appetite:** With your baby's growth accelerating, your body needs more nutrients. It's important to focus on a balanced diet that includes a variety of fruits, vegetables, whole grains, and lean proteins. Keep healthy snacks on hand to satisfy your hunger between meals.

Preparation Tips:

- **Talk to your baby:** Since your baby can now hear sounds, take the time to talk, sing, or read to them.

This can help strengthen the bond between you and your baby and may even be soothing to them.

- **Consider prenatal yoga:** Prenatal yoga can be an excellent way to relieve back pain, improve posture, and relax your mind. Look for classes specifically designed for pregnant women, or find a prenatal yoga video to follow at home.

- **Plan a babymoon:** If you're feeling up to it, now might be the perfect time to plan a relaxing getaway with your partner before the baby arrives. It's a great way to unwind and spend quality time together before your lives get even busier.

WEEK 19: MAJOR MILESTONES AND MOVEMENTS

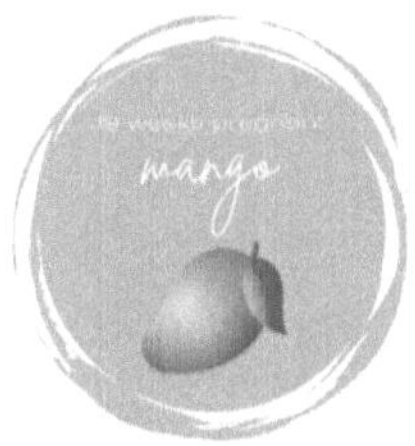

Baby's Size: A mango

Mother's Symptoms: Stretch marks, leg cramps, vivid dreams

What to Expect:

By week 19, your baby is the size of a mango and is becoming more active every day. Their arms and legs are in proportion to the rest of their body, and they're continuing to grow muscle. You might start to feel more distinct movements as your baby stretches, kicks, and flips inside the womb. The vernix caseosa, a waxy coating that protects your baby's skin from the amniotic fluid, is starting to form.

For you, the physical signs of pregnancy may become more visible as your belly expands and stretch marks begin to appear. A lot of ladies don't get these, which surprised me - I thought These silvery lines are a normal part of pregnancy as your skin stretches to accommodate your growing baby.

You might also experience leg cramps, particularly at night, and more vivid dreams due to hormonal changes.

More on the Symptoms You Might Experience This Week:

- **Stretch Marks:** Stretch marks are common during pregnancy and occur as your skin stretches rapidly. Keeping your skin moisturized can help reduce their appearance, though genetics also play a significant role. Remember, these marks are a testament to the incredible work your body is doing.
- **Leg Cramps:** Leg cramps, especially at night, are a common pregnancy complaint. They may be caused by the pressure of your growing uterus on the nerves and blood vessels that lead to your legs. Stretching before bed, staying hydrated, and wearing supportive shoes can help prevent them. And let's not forget regular walks!
- **Vivid Dreams:** Pregnancy hormones can lead to more intense and vivid dreams. These dreams are a normal part of pregnancy and often reflect your thoughts, fears, and anticipation about the changes ahead.

Preparation Tips:

- **Prepare for your anatomy scan:** Around week 20, you'll have your detailed anatomy scan. This is an exciting opportunity to see your baby in more detail and ensure that everything is developing as it should. If you're interested in finding out your baby's gender, now is the time to ask.

- **Gender Reveal**: Some people love to plan a unique way to reveal the gender of their baby. This can even be combined with a baby shower as then you can have what you need for baby much earlier so you're not down to the wire preparing. If you want to do a gender reveal party, plan it now so you are ready to do it (online or in person), when you have the results.

- **Start planning the nursery:** With your baby becoming more real by the day, this is a great time to start planning the nursery. Consider themes, colors, and essential furniture pieces. It's a fun and creative way to prepare for your baby's arrival.

- **Continue bonding with your baby:** Now that your baby can hear and move, continue talking, singing, and playing music. You can also involve your partner in these bonding activities to help them connect with the baby as well.

WEEK 20: THE HALFWAY MARK!

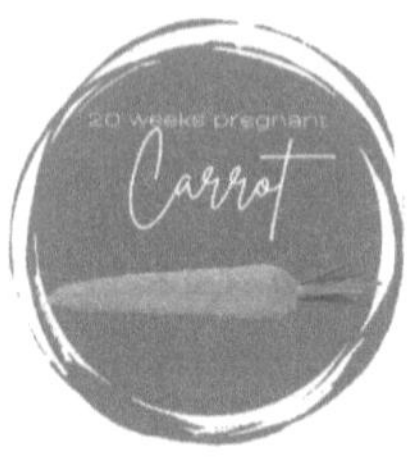

Baby's Size: A carrot

Mother's Symptoms: More pronounced baby movements, slight swelling, heartburn

What to Expect:

Congratulations momma-in-the-making!! You've reached the halfway point of your pregnancy! At week 20, your baby is about the size of a carrot and is growing rapidly. Their skin is developing, and they're starting to grow more hair on their head, eyebrows, and eyelashes. Inside, your baby's digestive system is developing, and they're beginning to produce meconium, their first bowel movement.

This is an exciting week for many moms-to-be because your baby's movements are becoming more pronounced. You might start to notice a pattern in their activity, with periods of sleep and wakefulness. However, with your growing baby, you might also experience some new symptoms, such as slight swelling in your feet and ankles and heartburn as your uterus presses on your stomach. From here forward, a pool super helps with the swelling if you have access to one.

I found that time crawled so slowly to the 20 weeks mark and then, as soon as I started the second half of my pregnancy, time went into superspeed. So buckle up!!

More on the Symptoms You Might Experience This Week:

- **More Pronounced Baby Movements:** Feeling your baby move is one of the most exciting parts of pregnancy. You may notice that they're more active at certain times of the day, especially when you're resting or after you've eaten. Enjoy these moments and take time to bond with your baby.
- **Slight Swelling:** Swelling, particularly in the feet and ankles, is common around this time as your body retains more fluid. To alleviate swelling, try to elevate your feet when sitting and avoid standing for long periods.
- **Heartburn:** Heartburn can be uncomfortable and is caused by your growing uterus putting pressure on your stomach. Eating smaller, more frequent meals, avoiding spicy or acidic foods, and not lying down right after eating can help reduce heartburn.

Preparation Tips:

- **Enjoy your anatomy scan:** This week or next, you'll have your detailed anatomy scan, where you can see your baby's development in detail. This is also when many parents find out their baby's gender, so be sure to let your healthcare provider know if you want to know.

- **Review your diet:** As heartburn and swelling become more common, it's a good idea to review your diet and make any necessary adjustments. Focus on nutrient-rich foods that support both your health and your baby's growth. Pro tip: delivery is harder when you're bigger than you need to be! Try not to overindulge, but if you do, give yourself some grace. It's not easy to eat right throughout a pregnancy!! We are all doing the best we can.

- **Document the halfway mark:** Reaching the halfway point is a big milestone! Consider documenting this moment with a photo of your baby bump or a special journal entry. It's a great way to celebrate how far you've come and look forward to the weeks ahead.

WEEK 21: SENSING THE WORLD

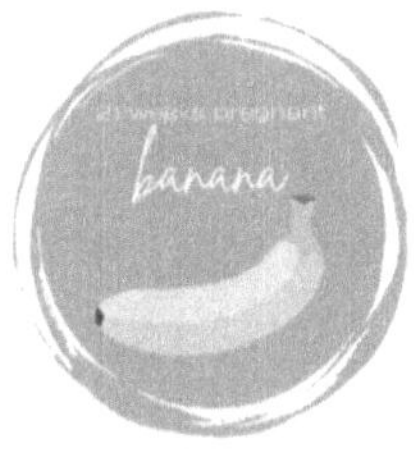

Baby's Size: A banana

Mother's Symptoms: Round ligament pain, varicose veins, increased energy

What to Expect:

At week 21, your baby is about the size of a banana and is becoming more aware of their surroundings. They're beginning to taste the amniotic fluid, which is influenced by the foods you eat, and their sense of touch is developing as they explore their environment by touching their face and body. Your baby's movements are likely becoming stronger, and you might even be able to feel them from the outside if you place your hand on your belly.

As your pregnancy progresses, you might experience round ligament pain more frequently, as well as varicose veins due to increased blood flow and pressure on your veins. However, many women find that their energy levels remain high during this time, making it a great opportunity to continue preparing for the baby's arrival.

More on the Symptoms You Might Experience This Week:

- **Round Ligament Pain:** This is a common discomfort as your uterus continues to grow and stretch the ligaments that support it. The pain is usually sharp and occurs when you move quickly or change positions. Moving slowly and using supportive pillows can help minimize discomfort.

- **Varicose Veins:** The increased blood flow during pregnancy, combined with the pressure from your growing uterus, can lead to varicose veins. Wearing compression stockings, elevating your legs, and avoiding prolonged standing can help reduce their appearance and discomfort.

- **Increased Energy:** Many women continue to experience high energy levels during the second trimester. Use this time to stay active, whether through walking, swimming, or prenatal exercise classes. It's also a great time to tackle projects at home, like organizing the nursery or preparing for the baby.

Preparation Tips:

- **Start discussing parental leave:** If you haven't already, start discussing parental leave with your employer. Make sure you understand your company's policies and begin planning how you'll manage your time off after the baby arrives.

- **Continue preparing the nursery:** With your energy levels up, continue working on the nursery. Start assembling furniture, organizing baby clothes, and decorating the space to make it cozy and welcoming. Pinterest was my BEST FRIEND for designing a nursery.

- **Involve your partner:** Pregnancy is a journey for both you and your partner. Involve them in bonding with the baby, preparing the nursery, and discussing plans for the future. It's a special time to connect and share in the excitement of what's to come.

Personal Story:

Amanda, who was 21 weeks pregnant, shared how she managed round ligament pain: "I started feeling sharp pains in my lower belly whenever I stood up too quickly or moved the wrong way. My doctor reassured me that it was just round ligament pain and nothing to worry about. I found that moving more slowly and using a pregnancy pillow for support really helped. It's just one of those things that comes with the territory, and I learned to be more mindful of how I moved to avoid the pain."

WEEK 22: BUILDING STRENGTH

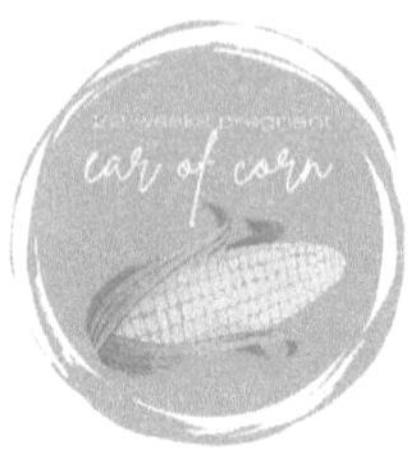

Baby's Size: An ear of corn

Mother's Symptoms: Swelling, backaches, vivid dreams

What to Expect:

At week 22, your baby is about the size of an ear of corn and is becoming stronger every day. Their muscles are developing, and they're starting to build up fat under their skin, which will help them regulate their body temperature after birth. Their bones are also hardening, and their grip is becoming more refined—your little one might even be able to grasp the umbilical cord. Additionally, your baby's senses are sharpening, and they're becoming more aware of the world around them, especially the sound of your voice.

For you, the physical changes of pregnancy continue. You might notice some swelling in your feet and ankles, particularly as the day goes on. Backaches are also common as your growing belly shifts your center of gravity and puts more strain on your back. Vivid dreams are another symptom many pregnant women experience, often a result of hormonal changes and the anticipation of becoming a parent.

Other Symptoms You Might Experience This Week:

- **Swelling**: Swelling in your feet and ankles is a common pregnancy symptom, especially after standing for long periods. To reduce swelling, try to elevate your feet whenever possible, wear comfortable shoes, and stay well-hydrated. Compression socks can also help improve circulation.

- **Backaches**: The added weight of your growing baby can cause backaches, especially in the lower back. Practice good posture, avoid lifting heavy objects, and consider prenatal yoga or gentle stretching to relieve discomfort. A warm bath or a heating pad can also provide relief.

- **Vivid Dreams**: Many women report having more intense and vivid dreams during pregnancy. This is likely due to a combination of hormonal changes, increased blood flow, and the emotional and psychological preparation for parenthood. If your dreams are unsettling, try relaxation techniques before bed, such as deep breathing or meditation.

Preparation Tips:

- **Continue talking to your baby**: Your baby's hearing is becoming more refined, so keep talking, singing, or playing music. This is a wonderful way to bond with your baby and helps them recognize your voice after birth.
- **Start planning your baby registry**: With your baby's arrival getting closer, now is a great time to start your baby registry. Consider the essentials you'll need, such as a crib, stroller, car seat, and baby clothes. It's also a fun way to involve family and friends in the preparations.
- **Focus on self-care**: With symptoms like backaches and swelling, it's important to prioritize self-care. Take time to rest, pamper yourself with a relaxing bath, and listen to your body's needs.

WEEK 23: GROWING SENSES AND STRONGER KICKS

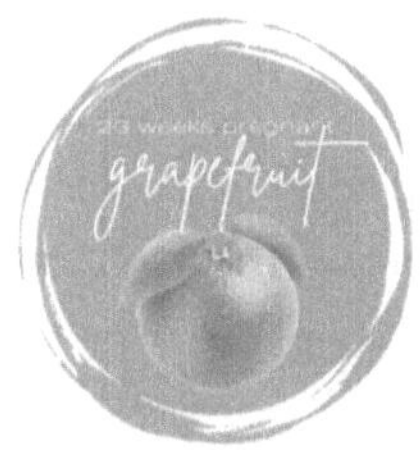

Baby's Size: A large grapefruit

Mother's Symptoms: Varicose veins, Braxton Hicks contractions, glowing skin

What to Expect:

At week 23, your baby is about the size of a large grapefruit and is continuing to develop at a rapid pace. Their sense of movement is well-developed, and they can feel you move as you go about your day. Your baby's hearing is also getting sharper, and they can distinguish between different types of sounds, including your heartbeat, your voice, and even loud noises outside the womb. Their kicks and movements are becoming stronger and more noticeable, providing constant reminders of their presence.

As your pregnancy progresses, you may notice the appearance of varicose veins, particularly in your legs. This is due to the increased blood volume and the pressure of your growing uterus on the veins in your lower body. You might also start experiencing Braxton Hicks contractions—mild, irregular contractions that are your body's way of preparing for labor. On the brighter side, many women continue to enjoy the "pregnancy glow," thanks to increased blood flow and hormonal changes that keep the skin looking radiant.

Other Symptoms You Might Experience This Week:

- Varicose Veins: Varicose veins can be uncomfortable and are caused by the increased pressure on your veins as your uterus grows. To minimize discomfort, avoid standing or sitting for long periods, elevate your legs when possible, and wear compression stockings to improve circulation.

- **Braxton Hicks Contractions**: These "practice" contractions are usually mild and irregular, and they help your uterus prepare for labor. If they become uncomfortable, try changing positions, drinking water, or practicing relaxation techniques like deep breathing.

- **Glowing Skin**: You probably still got that glow! The pregnancy glow is often attributed to increased blood circulation and hormonal changes that make your skin look more radiant. Enjoy this natural beauty boost, and take care of your skin with gentle, hydrating products.

Preparation Tips:

- **Stay active**: Regular exercise, such as walking or swimming, can help prevent varicose veins and manage other pregnancy symptoms. Staying active also boosts your energy levels and helps you maintain a healthy weight.

- **Monitor Braxton Hicks contractions**: While Braxton Hicks contractions are normal, it's important to distinguish them from true labor contractions. If you notice a pattern or if they become more intense, contact your healthcare provider.

- **Continue working on the nursery**: With your baby's arrival approaching, continue to prepare the nursery. Start assembling furniture, organizing baby clothes, and adding decorative touches to make the space warm and inviting.

WEEK 24: VIABILITY AND VITAL DEVELOPMENTS

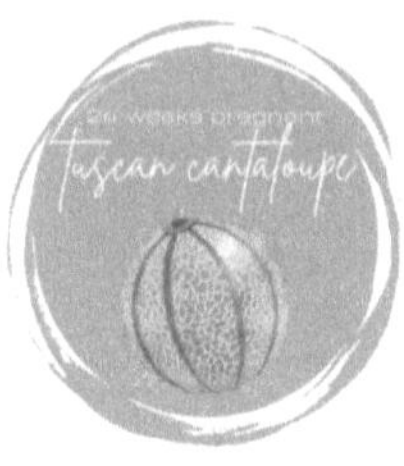

Baby's Size: A Tuscan cantaloupe

Mother's Symptoms: Increased appetite, heartburn, sensitive gums

What to Expect:

At week 24, your baby is about the size of a Tucan cantaloupe and is now considered "viable," meaning they have a chance of survival outside the womb with medical support if born prematurely. This is a significant milestone in your pregnancy. You are now officially at the point where if your baby needed to be born, it could survive. Your baby's lungs are developing branches of the respiratory tree and cells that produce surfactant, which will help their lungs inflate with air after birth. Their brain is growing rapidly, and they're continuing to gain weight and muscle mass.

For you, your growing baby might be making you feel hungrier than ever as your body demands more energy.

However, this increased appetite might also bring along heartburn, as your expanding uterus puts pressure on your stomach. Another common symptom during this time is sensitive gums, which can bleed more easily due to hormonal changes.

More on the Symptoms You Might Experience This Week:

- **Increased Appetite**: Your baby's growth is accelerating, and so is your appetite. Focus on nutrient-rich foods that support both you and your baby. Eating smaller, more frequent meals can help manage hunger and keep your energy levels stable.

- **Heartburn**: Heartburn is a common complaint during the second trimester, caused by your growing uterus pressing on your stomach. To reduce heartburn, avoid spicy or acidic foods, eat smaller meals, and try not to lie down immediately after eating.

- **Sensitive Gums**: Hormonal changes can make your gums more sensitive and prone to bleeding. Maintain good oral hygiene by brushing and flossing regularly, and consider using a soft-bristled toothbrush to reduce irritation.

Preparation Tips:

- **Prepare for your glucose screening**: Between weeks 24-28, you'll have a glucose screening test to check for gestational diabetes. Talk to your healthcare provider about what to expect and how to prepare for the test.
- **Update your wardrobe**: As your belly continues to grow, you might need to update your maternity wardrobe. Look for comfortable, stretchy clothing that can accommodate your changing shape.
- **Start thinking about childcare**: If you plan to return to work after your baby is born, now is a good time to start researching childcare options. Whether you're considering daycare, a nanny, or family support, it's important to plan ahead.

WEEK 25: GETTING READY FOR THE FINAL STRETCH

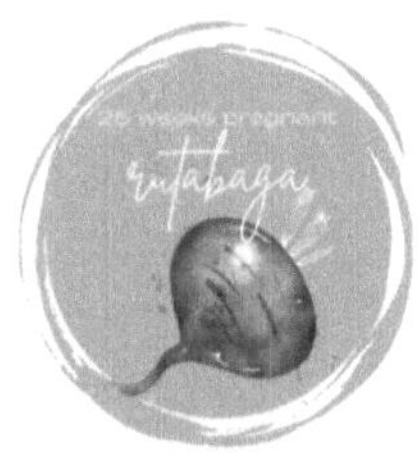

Baby's Size: A rutabaga

Mother's Symptoms: Shortness of breath, backaches, itchy skin

What to Expect:

At week 25, your baby is about the size of a rutabaga and is continuing to grow and develop in preparation for the final trimester. Their lungs are developing further, and their nostrils, which were previously closed, are beginning to open, allowing them to start practicing breathing by inhaling amniotic fluid. Your baby's skin is gradually becoming less translucent as they gain more fat, and their hair continues to grow.

As your baby grows, you might experience shortness of breath as your expanding uterus pushes against your diaphragm, making it harder to take deep breaths. Backaches are also common as your body adjusts to the extra weight. Additionally, you might notice that your skin feels itchier than usual, especially around your belly as it stretches to accommodate your growing baby.

More on the Symptoms You Might Experience This Week:

- **Shortness of Breath**: As your baby grows and your uterus expands, it can become more difficult to take deep breaths. Try to sit or stand up straight to give your lungs more room to expand, and take breaks to catch your breath when needed.
- **Backaches**: The weight of your growing baby can put extra strain on your back, leading to discomfort. Consider using a maternity support belt to alleviate pressure on your lower back, and practice gentle stretches to relieve tension.
- **Itchy Skin**: As your skin stretches to accommodate your growing belly, it might become dry and itchy. Keep your skin hydrated with a good moisturizer, and avoid hot showers, which can strip your skin of its natural oils.

Preparation Tips:

- **Begin planning your maternity leave**: If you haven't already, now is a good time to start planning your maternity leave. Make sure you understand your company's policies and discuss your plans with your employer.

- **Prepare for Braxton Hicks contractions**: As you approach the third trimester, Braxton Hicks contractions may become more frequent. Practice relaxation techniques, such as deep breathing or visualization, to help you manage these contractions.

- **Stay active and listen to your body**: Regular physical activity, such as walking or swimming, can help keep you fit and reduce discomfort. However, it's important to listen to your body and rest when needed. Don't push yourself too hard—your body is already working hard to support your growing baby.

Personal Story:

Olivia, who was 25 weeks pregnant, shared how she managed shortness of breath: "I started noticing that I was getting winded much more easily, especially when going up stairs or doing anything active. My doctor reassured me that this was normal as my baby was taking up more space. I found that taking breaks, sitting up straight, and focusing on my breathing really helped. It was a good reminder to slow down and take things easy as I prepared for the final trimester."

WEEK 26: PREPARING FOR THE FINAL STRETCH

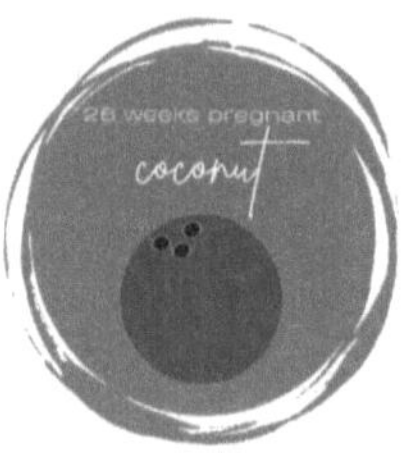

Baby's Size: A coconut

Mother's Symptoms: Shortness of breath, Braxton Hicks contractions, trouble sleeping

What to Expect:

At week 26, your baby is about the size of a coconut and is preparing for the final stages of development. Their eyes are starting to open, and they're practicing blinking. The lungs are continuing to mature, and your baby is beginning to make breathing movements, although they're still inhaling amniotic fluid rather than air. Your baby's brain is also developing rapidly, creating more complex neural connections.

As your baby grows, you might notice that breathing becomes a bit more challenging. This is due to your expanding uterus pressing against your diaphragm, making it harder to take deep breaths. Additionally, you might start experiencing Braxton Hicks contractions, which are mild, irregular contractions that help your body prepare for labor. Trouble sleeping is also common as your belly grows and it becomes harder to find a comfortable position.

Other Symptoms You Might Experience This Week:

- **Shortness of Breath:** As your baby takes up more space, it can become harder to breathe deeply. Try sitting or standing up straight to give your lungs more room to expand, and practice deep breathing exercises to improve lung capacity. Sleeping with your upper body elevated can also help.

- **Braxton Hicks Contractions:** These "practice" contractions are usually mild and irregular but can sometimes be uncomfortable. They're your body's way of preparing for labor. If the contractions become painful or regular, it's important to contact your healthcare provider. They may have started a few weeks ago for you or you may have noticed the first one this week.

- **Trouble Sleeping:** Finding a comfortable sleeping position can be challenging as your belly grows. All you belly sleepers out there, I feel you!! Obviously that's out until after pregnancy or maybe never ☺ Consider using a pregnancy pillow to support your belly and back, and try sleeping on your side with your knees bent. Creating a bedtime routine and avoiding heavy meals before bed can also improve your sleep quality.

Preparation Tips:

- **Growth Ultrasound:** If your healthcare provider recommends it, a growth ultrasound around this time can help ensure that your baby is developing as expected. It's also a great opportunity to see your baby and get an update on their progress.

- **Prepare for Maternity Leave:** Now is a good time to finalize your plans for maternity leave. Make sure you have all the necessary paperwork in order and discuss your plans with your employer. Preparing ahead of time will help you feel more relaxed as your due date approaches.

- **Plan Your Baby Shower:** If you haven't already, now is the perfect time to finalize the details of your baby shower. Whether it's a big party or a small gathering, it's a wonderful opportunity to celebrate your pregnancy with loved ones and gather essentials for your baby. If you are someone that is very particular about what you want in your nursery and so you'd rather not have people gift you things that are the wrong color and size, consider a fund for your baby shower! I had a "diaper fund" so everyone brought diapers. I also had a post-partum doula fund because I knew I wanted that help and I didn't have the budget for it. Just some ideas! This is your pregnancy and you can really do whatever you want, so plan the baby shower and registry list that works for you. In the free e-book that I gave you at the beginning of this book I include 10 things that I love the MOST of all baby purchases out there. Take a look and see if any of them are a good fit for your registry.

WEEK 27: ENTERING THE THIRD TRIMESTER

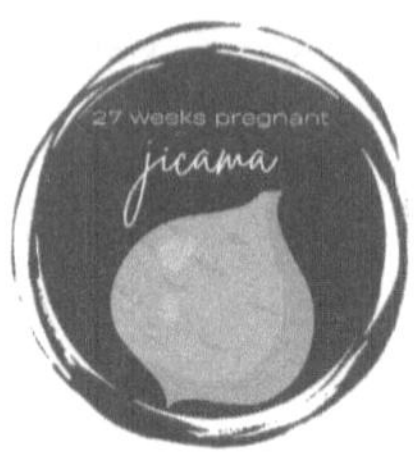

Baby's Size: A jicama

Mother's Symptoms: Heartburn, lots of baby kicks, swelling

What to Expect:

Welcome to week 27, the final week of your second trimester! Your baby is now about the size of a jicama and is continuing to grow and develop rapidly. Their lungs are maturing, and they're practicing more complex movements like sucking and swallowing, which will be essential after birth. Your baby's sleep-wake cycles are becoming more established, and you might notice patterns in their movements.

As you near the third trimester, some symptoms might become more pronounced. Heartburn can be more frequent as your growing uterus pushes on your stomach, making it easier for stomach acid to escape into your esophagus. Your baby's movements are likely stronger and more noticeable, and you might even see your belly move as they kick and roll. Swelling, particularly in your feet and ankles, is also common as your body retains more fluids.

Other Symptoms You Might Experience This Week:

- **Heartburn:** Heartburn is common during pregnancy due to the relaxation of the valve between your stomach and esophagus caused by pregnancy hormones. Eating smaller, more frequent meals, avoiding spicy or acidic foods, and not lying down immediately after eating can help manage heartburn. Talk to your healthcare provider about safe antacids if needed.

- **Lots of Baby Kicks:** Your baby's movements are becoming stronger and more coordinated. These kicks and rolls are reassuring signs that your baby is healthy and active. Keep track of their movements, as it can be an important indicator of their well-being. If you notice a decrease in movement, contact your healthcare provider.

- **Swelling:** Swelling in your feet and ankles is common during the third trimester due to increased fluid retention and the pressure of your growing uterus on your veins. Elevating your feet, wearing comfortable shoes, and staying hydrated can help reduce swelling. Avoid standing or sitting for long periods when possible.

Preparation Tips:

- **Rhogam Shot:** If you're Rh-negative, your provider will likely recommend a Rhogam shot around this time to prevent complications with your baby's blood type. This is a routine and important part of prenatal care, so be sure to discuss it with your healthcare provider.
- **Consider Childbirth Classes:** As you approach the third trimester, it's a good idea to start thinking about childbirth classes. These classes can provide valuable information on labor, delivery, and newborn care, helping you feel more prepared and confident.
- **Continue Bonding with Your Baby:** Now that your baby's movements are more pronounced, continue talking, singing, or reading to them. This is a special way to bond with your baby and helps them become familiar with your voice.

Personal Story:

Lydia, who was 27 weeks pregnant, shared her experience with heartburn: "Heartburn became my constant companion as I approached the third trimester. It seemed like no matter what I ate, I would feel that burning sensation afterward. I found that eating smaller meals more frequently and avoiding anything too spicy or acidic really helped. My doctor also suggested sleeping with my upper body slightly elevated, which made a huge difference at night. It's just one of those things you learn to manage, and it was comforting to know it was a normal part of pregnancy. And even more comforting to know it will subside after pregnancy!"

THIRD TRIMESTER (WEEKS 28-40+)

WEEK 28: WELCOME TO THE THIRD TRIMESTER

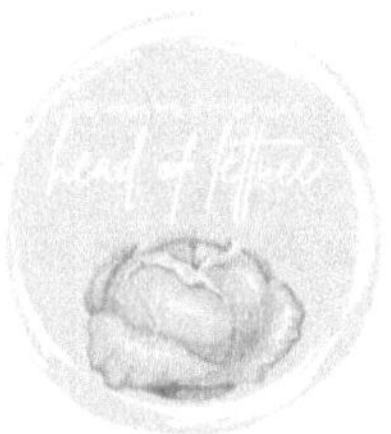

Baby's Size: A head of lettuce

Mother's Symptoms: Sleep troubles, Braxton Hicks contractions, more frequent kicks

What to Expect:

Welcome to week 28, the start of your third trimester! Your baby is now about the size of a head of lettuce and is gearing up for the final weeks of growth and development. At this stage, your baby's brain is developing rapidly, and their eyes can open and close. They're also continuing to gain weight, and you might notice stronger and more frequent movements as your baby stretches and practices kicking.

As your baby grows, you might experience more difficulty sleeping due to your expanding belly and increased activity from your little one. Braxton Hicks contractions may become more noticeable, as your body prepares for labor. These "practice" contractions are typically mild and irregular, but they can sometimes be uncomfortable. You'll also likely notice that your baby's movements are more pronounced, with kicks that can sometimes catch you by surprise!

Other Symptoms You Might Experience This Week:

- **Sleep Troubles**: Finding a comfortable position can be a challenge as your belly grows. Consider using a pregnancy pillow to support your back, belly, and hips. Sleeping on your left side can improve circulation and may help you rest more comfortably.

- **Braxton Hicks Contractions**: These contractions are your body's way of preparing for labor. They're usually not painful and can be relieved by changing positions, drinking water, or practicing relaxation techniques. If they become regular or painful, contact your healthcare provider.

- **Frequent Kicks:** Your baby's kicks and movements are a reassuring sign that they're healthy and active. Take time to enjoy these moments and consider doing kick counts to track your baby's activity.

Preparation Tips:

- **Begin kick counts**: Your healthcare provider may recommend tracking your baby's movements to ensure they're staying active. Set aside time each day to count how many kicks, rolls, or other movements you feel within a set period.

- **Start packing your hospital bag**: With your due date approaching, it's a good idea to start packing your hospital bag. Include essentials like comfortable clothing, toiletries, and any items you'll want during labor and your hospital stay.

- **Update your birth plan:** If you have a birth plan, now is a good time to review and update it. Consider discussing your preferences with your healthcare provider and ensuring your support person is familiar with your plan.

WEEK 29: BABY'S SENSES ARE SHARPENING

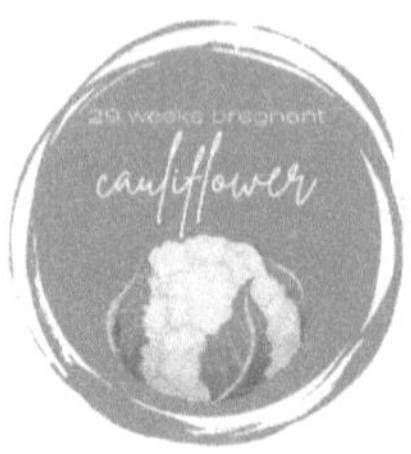

Baby's Size: A head of cauliflower

Mother's Symptoms: Frequent bathroom trips, backaches, varicose veins

What to Expect:

At week 29, your baby is about the size of a head of cauliflower and is becoming more aware of the world around them. Their senses are sharpening, and they can now react to light, sound, and touch. Your baby's muscles and lungs continue to mature, and they're practicing movements like sucking and breathing in preparation for life outside the womb.

As your baby grows, you'll likely notice an increase in frequent bathroom trips as your baby presses on your bladder. Backaches are also common due to the extra weight you're carrying, and varicose veins may become more pronounced as your circulation works harder to support both you and your baby. While these symptoms can be uncomfortable, they're normal parts of pregnancy.

Other Symptoms You Might Experience This Week:

- **Frequent Bathroom Trips**: With your growing baby putting pressure on your bladder, you might find yourself needing to use the bathroom more often. Stay hydrated but try to limit fluids before bedtime to reduce nighttime trips.

- **Backaches**: The added weight and shifting center of gravity can cause back pain. Practice good posture, consider using a maternity support belt, and try gentle stretching or prenatal yoga to relieve discomfort.

- **Varicose Veins**: Varicose veins can appear as your blood volume increases and circulation slows. Wearing compression stockings, elevating your legs when sitting, and avoiding long periods of standing can help reduce discomfort.

Preparation Tips:

- **Prepare for the glucose screening test**: If you haven't had your glucose screening test yet, it will likely happen around this time. This test checks for gestational diabetes and is an important part of prenatal care.

- **Continue setting up the nursery**: As you approach the final weeks of pregnancy, continue working on the nursery. Make sure the crib is assembled, and all essential items, such as diapers and baby clothes, are ready for your baby's arrival.

- **Focus on comfort**: With backaches and bathroom trips increasing, it's important to focus on your comfort. Invest in supportive shoes, comfortable clothing, and take breaks throughout the day to rest and recharge. If you have access to a pool it is so nice to swim and really good for your joints and swelling.

WEEK 30: BABY IS PRACTICING BREATHING

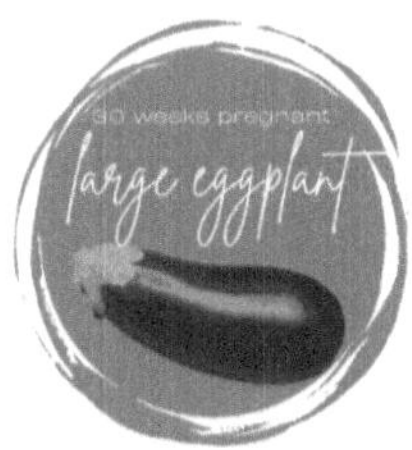

Baby's Size: A large eggplant

Mother's Symptoms: Fatigue, heartburn, swollen feet

What to Expect:

At week 30, your baby is about the size of a large eggplant and is continuing to gain weight and strength. Their lungs are maturing, and they're practicing breathing movements by inhaling and exhaling amniotic fluid. Your baby's brain is also growing rapidly, and their body is beginning to store more fat, which will help regulate their body temperature after birth.

As your baby grows, you might start to feel more fatigued as your body works harder to support both you and your baby. Heartburn can be more frequent as your expanding uterus puts pressure on your stomach. Swelling in your feet and ankles is also common due to increased fluid retention and the pressure of your growing baby on your veins.

More on the Symptoms You Might Experience This Week:

- **Fatigue**: As you enter the final weeks of pregnancy, fatigue may return. Listen to your body and rest when you need to. It's important to conserve your energy for labor and delivery.

- **Heartburn**: Heartburn is common in the third trimester as your baby pushes your stomach upwards. Eating smaller, more frequent meals, avoiding spicy or acidic foods, and not lying down immediately after eating can help reduce heartburn.

- **Swollen Feet**: Swelling, especially in your feet and ankles, is a normal part of pregnancy. Elevating your feet, staying hydrated, and wearing comfortable shoes can help manage swelling. If the swelling is severe or sudden, contact your healthcare provider.

Preparation Tips:

- **Plan for postpartum care**: As you prepare for your baby's arrival, start thinking about your postpartum care. Stock up on essentials like pads, comfortable clothing, and any items you'll need for recovery.

- **Practice relaxation techniques**: As you approach the final weeks of pregnancy, practicing relaxation techniques can help you manage stress and prepare for labor. Consider deep breathing exercises, meditation, or prenatal yoga.

- **Monitor your baby's movements**: Continue to track your baby's movements and contact your healthcare provider if you notice any significant changes. Regular movement is a sign that your baby is healthy and active.

WEEK 31: GETTING READY FOR THE BIG DAY

Baby's Size: A pineapple

Mother's Symptoms: General discomfort, Braxton Hicks contractions, leaky breasts

What to Expect:

At week 31, your baby is about the size of a pineapple and is preparing for their big debut. They're continuing to gain weight, and their bones are hardening, although the skull remains soft and flexible to make it easier for them to pass through the birth canal. Your baby's brain and nervous system are also developing rapidly, and their five senses are now fully functional.

As your due date approaches, you might experience general discomfort as your body prepares for labor. Braxton Hicks contractions may become more frequent, and you might notice that your breasts are starting to leak colostrum, the nutrient-rich fluid that will feed your baby in the first few days after birth. These changes are all signs that your body is getting ready for the final stretch.

Other Symptoms You Might Experience This Week:

- **General Discomfort**: As your baby takes up more space, you might feel a general sense of discomfort, especially in your back, hips, and abdomen. Practice good posture, use supportive pillows, and take breaks throughout the day to rest.

- **Braxton Hicks Contractions**: These "practice" contractions may become more noticeable and frequent as your body prepares for labor. If they become regular or painful, contact your healthcare provider.

- **Leaky Breasts**: It's normal for your breasts to start leaking colostrum as they prepare for breastfeeding. Wearing breast pads can help absorb any leaks and keep you comfortable.

Preparation Tips:

- **Start thinking about your birth plan**: If you haven't already, now is a good time to finalize your birth plan. Consider your preferences for labor and delivery, and discuss them with your healthcare provider.

- **Pack your hospital bag**: Make sure your hospital bag is packed and ready to go. Include essentials like comfortable clothing, toiletries, and any items you'll need during labor and your hospital stay.

- **Stay hydrated and nourished**: As you approach the final weeks of pregnancy, it's important to stay hydrated and nourished. Focus on eating nutrient-rich foods and drinking plenty of water to support both you and your baby.

Personal Story:

Monica, who was 31 weeks pregnant, shared how she managed Braxton Hicks contractions: "The Braxton Hicks contractions started getting stronger around week 31, and at first, I was worried I was going into labor. But after talking to my doctor, I learned they were just practice contractions. I found that drinking water and changing positions helped, and I tried to use them as an opportunity to practice my breathing techniques for labor. It was reassuring to know my body was getting ready for the big day."

WEEK 32: BABY'S POSITIONING AND PREPARING FOR BIRTH

Baby's Size: A butternut squash

Mother's Symptoms: Pelvic pressure, shortness of breath, leaky breasts

What to Expect:

At week 32, your baby is about the size of a butternut squash and is likely settling into a head-down position, preparing for birth. They're practicing essential skills like sucking, breathing, and swallowing, and their bones are fully developed, though still soft enough for delivery. Your baby's skin is also becoming smoother as they continue to gain fat, which will help regulate their body temperature after birth.

As your baby moves lower into your pelvis, you might feel increased pelvic pressure, a sign that your body is preparing for labor. You might also experience shortness of breath as your expanding uterus presses on your diaphragm, making it harder to take deep breaths. Additionally, your breasts might start leaking colostrum, the first form of milk that will nourish your baby in the early days after birth.

Other Symptoms You Might Experience This Week:

- **Pelvic Pressure**: The pressure in your pelvis is a sign that your baby is moving into position for birth. This pressure, known as "lightening," can cause discomfort, but it's also a positive sign that your body is preparing for labor. Walking and gentle exercises can help alleviate some of the discomfort.
- **Shortness of Breath**: As your baby grows, your diaphragm has less room to expand, which can make breathing more difficult. Try to sit up straight and take slow, deep breaths to improve lung capacity. Sleeping with your upper body elevated can also help reduce shortness of breath at night.
- **Leaky Breasts**: It's common for your breasts to start leaking colostrum as they prepare for breastfeeding. Wearing breast pads inside your bra can help absorb leaks and keep you comfortable.

Preparation Tips:

- **Install the Car Seat**: Now is the time to install your baby's car seat and ensure it's properly fitted. You can have it checked by a certified car seat technician for added peace of mind.

- **Finalize Your Birth Plan**: Review your birth plan with your healthcare provider and make any final adjustments. Discuss your preferences for labor, pain management, and postpartum care, and ensure your support person is familiar with your plan.

- **Start Packing Your Hospital Bag**: It's a good idea to start packing your hospital bag with essentials like comfortable clothing, toiletries, and items you'll need during labor and your hospital stay. Don't forget to pack some snacks and a phone charger!

WEEK 33: NESTING INSTINCTS AND PREPARING FOR LABOR

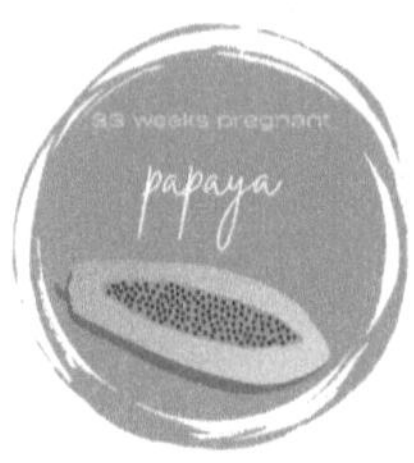

Baby's Size: A papaya

Mother's Symptoms: Intense Braxton Hicks, nesting urges, back pain

What to Expect:

At week 33, your baby is about the size of a papaya and is continuing to grow and develop rapidly. Their lungs are almost fully mature, and they're practicing breathing movements in preparation for their first breath after birth. Your baby's brain and nervous system are also developing, and they're becoming more sensitive to light and sound.

You might start to notice that Braxton Hicks contractions are becoming more frequent and intense as your body gears up for labor. These "practice" contractions are usually irregular and not painful, but they can be uncomfortable. The nesting instinct might also kick in strongly, giving you the urge to clean, organize, and prepare your home for your baby's arrival. Additionally, back pain is common as your body supports your growing baby.

Other Symptoms You Might Experience This Week:

- **Intense Braxton Hicks**: These contractions are a normal part of pregnancy and help your body prepare for labor. They're usually irregular and can be relieved by changing positions, drinking water, or resting. If they become regular or painful, contact your healthcare provider.

- **Nesting Urges**: The nesting instinct is a powerful urge to prepare your home for your baby's arrival. While it's natural to want everything to be perfect, be sure to listen to your body and not overdo it. Take breaks and delegate tasks when possible.

- **Back Pain**: Back pain is common in the third trimester due to the extra weight you're carrying. Consider using a maternity support belt, practicing good posture, and doing gentle stretches or prenatal yoga to relieve discomfort.

Preparation Tips:

- **Complete Last-Minute Shopping**: Make sure you have all the essentials for your baby's arrival, including diapers, wipes, and baby clothes. It's also a good time to stock up on postpartum supplies for yourself, such as pads, nursing bras, and comfortable clothing.

- **Plan for Postpartum Support**: Think about what kind of support you'll need after your baby arrives. Arrange for help with meals, household chores, and childcare for older children. Having a support system in place will allow you to focus on recovering and bonding with your baby.

- **Practice Relaxation Techniques**: As you prepare for labor, practice relaxation techniques such as deep breathing, visualization, or meditation. These can help you stay calm and focused during labor and delivery.

WEEK 34: BABY DROPPING AND FINAL PREPARATIONS

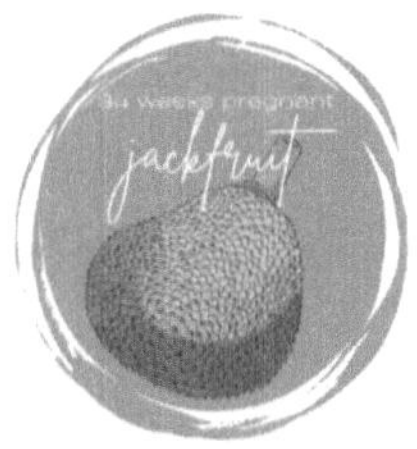

Baby's Size: A jackfruit

Mother's Symptoms: Pelvic pressure, swelling, fatigue

What to Expect:

At week 34, your baby is about the size of a jackfruit and is likely dropping lower into your pelvis in preparation for birth. This process, known as "lightening," can cause increased pelvic pressure, but it also means that your baby is getting ready for their big debut. Your baby's immune system is developing, and they're continuing to gain weight and build up fat stores to help regulate their body temperature after birth.

As your baby drops, you might experience more noticeable pelvic pressure and discomfort. Swelling, especially in your feet and ankles, is also common as your body retains more fluid. Fatigue may return as your body works hard to support both you and your growing baby during these final weeks.

Other Symptoms You Might Experience This Week:

- **Pelvic Pressure**: As your baby moves lower into your pelvis, you might feel increased pressure and discomfort. Walking and gentle stretches can help ease some of the pressure. A maternity support belt can also provide additional support and alleviate discomfort.

- **Swelling**: Swelling in your feet and ankles is a common symptom in the third trimester. To reduce swelling, try to elevate your feet whenever possible, stay hydrated, and avoid standing or sitting for long periods. Compression socks can also help improve circulation. From this week forward the swelling in your ankles and wrists could cause carpal tunnel syndrome and something similar for your feet. My good friend couldn't hold a spoon in her hand in the morning for the last month of her pregnancy as her fingers were totally numb in the mornings! I had this too, to a degree, but not like that. If this happens, you can run cold water over your wrists at night before bed and wear a compression bandage. Also you can wear a splint at night to keep your wrists neutral.

- **Fatigue**: As you approach the end of your pregnancy, fatigue may return. Listen to your body and rest when you need to. It's important to conserve your energy for labor and delivery.

Preparation Tips:

- **Install the Car Seat**: If you haven't already, make sure your baby's car seat is installed and properly fitted. Many hospitals require you to have a car seat before they'll let you leave with your baby.

- **Finalize the Nursery**: Make sure the nursery is fully set up and stocked with everything you'll need for your baby's arrival. This includes having the crib assembled, diapers and wipes on hand, and baby clothes washed and ready.

- **Prepare for the Group B Strep Test**: Around week 35-37, your healthcare provider will likely perform a Group B Strep test to check for this common bacteria. If you test positive, you'll receive antibiotics during labor to protect your baby.

WEEK 35: THE HOME STRETCH

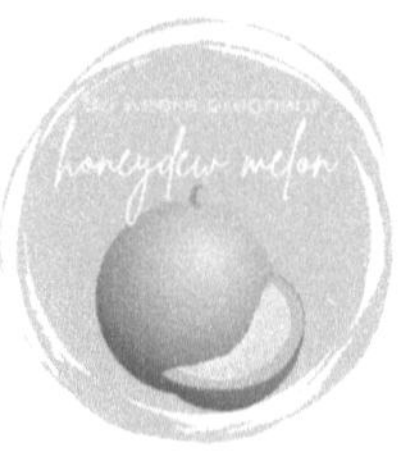

Baby's Size: A honeydew melon

Mother's Symptoms: More frequent Braxton Hicks, increased discharge, nesting instinct

What to Expect:

At week 35, your baby is about the size of a honeydew melon and is continuing to prepare for life outside the womb. Their lungs are fully developed, and they're gaining about half a pound a week as they build up fat stores that will help regulate their body temperature after birth. Your baby's movements may feel different now as they run out of room, but they should still be active.

As your body prepares for labor, you might notice more frequent Braxton Hicks contractions, increased vaginal discharge, and an even stronger nesting instinct. These are all signs that your body is getting ready for the big day. It's an exciting time, but it can also be overwhelming as you prepare for the arrival of your little one.

More on the Symptoms You Might Experience This Week:

- **More Frequent Braxton Hicks**: These practice contractions may become more frequent as your body prepares for labor. If they become regular or painful, it's important to contact your healthcare provider, as it could be a sign of early labor.

- **Increased Discharge**: It's common to experience an increase in vaginal discharge as you approach the end of your pregnancy. This is your body's way of preparing for labor. If you notice a sudden increase or if the discharge is watery, it's important to contact your healthcare provider.

- **Nesting Instinct**: The nesting instinct may be in full swing, and you might feel a strong urge to clean, organize, and prepare your home for your baby's arrival. While it's natural to want everything to be perfect, be sure to listen to your body and not overdo it.

Preparation Tips:

- **Finalize Your Hospital Bag**: Make sure your hospital bag is packed and ready to go. Include essentials like comfortable clothing, toiletries, and any items you'll need during labor and your hospital stay. Don't forget to pack some snacks and a phone charger!

- **Review Your Birth Plan**: Review your birth plan with your healthcare provider and make sure your support person is familiar with it. Consider any last-minute adjustments you might want to make.

- **Plan for Postpartum Support**: Think about what kind of support you'll need after your baby arrives. Arrange for help with meals, household chores, and childcare for older children. Having a support system in place will allow you to focus on recovering and bonding with your baby. If you went with a postpartum doula make sure that stuff is all scheduled!

Personal Story:

Emily, who was 35 weeks pregnant, shared her experience with nesting: "At 35 weeks, I was in full-on nesting mode. I wanted everything to be perfect for the baby, from organizing the nursery to making sure the house was spotless. It gave me a sense of control and helped me feel prepared for the big day. But I also had to remind myself to take breaks and not push too hard. It was all about finding balance and getting ready for the amazing journey ahead."

WEEK 36: PREPARING FOR THE FINAL COUNTDOWN

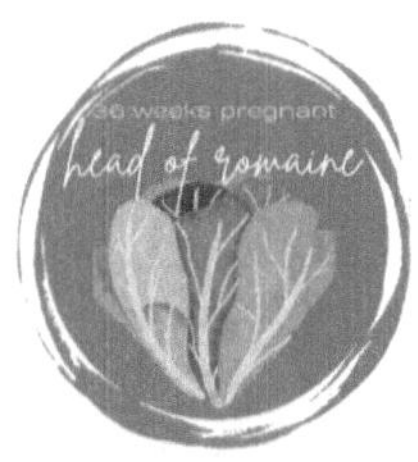

Baby's Size: A head of romaine lettuce

Mother's Symptoms: Pelvic discomfort, frequent urination, Braxton Hicks contractions

What to Expect:

At week 36, your baby is about the size of a head of romaine lettuce and is settling into the final stages of development. They're continuing to gain weight, and their organs are fully mature, including the lungs, which are now ready to support breathing after birth. Your baby is likely in the head-down position, preparing for delivery, and may drop lower into your pelvis, a process we mentioned last week, known as "lightening."

As your baby moves into position, you might feel increased pelvic discomfort and pressure. This is a common symptom as your baby's head presses against your pelvis. You'll also likely experience more frequent urination as your baby puts pressure on your bladder. Braxton Hicks contractions may become more frequent and intense as your body gears up for labor. These "practice" contractions are irregular and usually not painful but can be uncomfortable.

More on the Symptoms You Might Experience This Week:
(A lot of these of symptoms continuing over from last week!)

- **Pelvic Discomfort**: As your baby drops lower into your pelvis, you may feel increased pressure and discomfort. This can make walking, standing, and sitting more uncomfortable. Gentle stretching, sitting on a birthing ball, and warm baths can help alleviate some of the pressure.

- **Frequent Urination**: The added pressure on your bladder from your baby's head may cause you to visit the bathroom more often. Stay hydrated, but consider limiting fluids in the evening to reduce nighttime trips to the bathroom.

- **Braxton Hicks Contractions**: These contractions are your body's way of preparing for labor. They're usually irregular and not as intense as real contractions. Changing positions, drinking water, or resting can help relieve Braxton Hicks contractions.

Preparation Tips:

- **Cervical Checks**: Your healthcare provider may begin checking your cervix for dilation and effacement, which are signs that labor is approaching. These checks can give you an idea of how close you are to delivery, but it's important to remember that every pregnancy is different, and progress varies.

- **Pack Your Hospital Bag**: Make sure your hospital bag is packed and ready to go. Include essentials like comfortable clothing, toiletries, and any items you'll need during labor and your hospital stay. Don't forget to pack snacks and a phone charger!

- **Discuss Labor Signs**: Review the signs of labor with your healthcare provider, including what to do if your water breaks or if you experience regular contractions. Knowing what to expect can help you feel more prepared and confident as your due date approaches.

WEEK 37: FULL-TERM AND READY TO GO

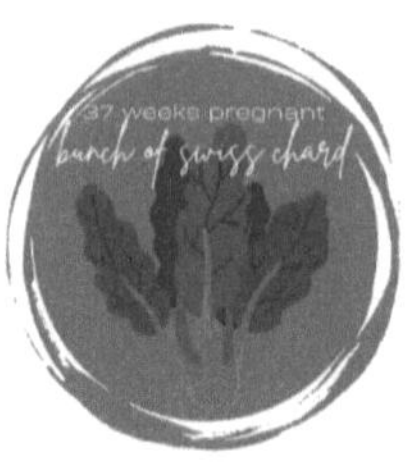

Baby's Size: A bunch of Swiss chard

Mother's Symptoms: Loss of mucus plug, nesting instinct, swelling

What to Expect:

Congratulations! At week 37, your baby is considered full-term and is about the size of a bunch of Swiss chard. They're fully developed and just about ready to make their grand entrance. Your baby is continuing to gain weight, and their brain and lungs are still maturing, even in these final weeks. They're also shedding the vernix caseosa, the waxy coating that has protected their skin during pregnancy.

You might notice some significant changes in your body as labor approaches. One key sign is the loss of your mucus plug, which is a thick collection of mucus that seals the cervix during pregnancy. Losing the mucus plug can be an indication that labor is near, although it doesn't always mean labor will start immediately. You may also experience a strong nesting instinct, urging you to clean and prepare your home for your baby's arrival. Swelling, particularly in your feet and ankles, may be more noticeable as your body retains more fluid.

Other Symptoms You Might Experience This Week:

- **Loss of Mucus Plug**: The mucus plug is a protective barrier that seals the cervix during pregnancy. Losing it can be a sign that labor is approaching, but it's not always immediate. It can happen days or even weeks before labor begins. If you notice a significant loss of mucus, especially if it's tinged with blood (known as a "bloody show"), contact your healthcare provider.

- **Nesting Instinct**: The urge to clean, organize, and prepare your home can be overwhelming as your due date approaches. While it's natural to want everything to be perfect, be careful not to overexert yourself, momma! Take breaks and prioritize tasks that will make you feel most prepared.

- **Swelling**: Swelling, particularly in your feet and ankles, is common in the final weeks of pregnancy. To reduce swelling, elevate your feet whenever possible, stay hydrated, and wear comfortable shoes. Compression stockings can also help improve circulation.

Preparation Tips:

- **Finalize Your Birth Plan**: Make sure your birth plan is finalized and shared with your healthcare provider. Consider any last-minute adjustments you might want to make, and ensure your support person is familiar with your preferences.

- **Prepare a Postpartum Care Kit**: Start gathering essentials for your postpartum recovery, such as pads, pain relief, and comfortable clothing. Items like a peri bottle, witch hazel pads, and a nursing pillow can make the postpartum period more comfortable.

- **Rest and Conserve Energy**: As your due date approaches, it's important to rest and conserve your energy for labor. While nesting is a common urge, make sure to balance your activity with plenty of rest.

WEEK 38: ON THE EDGE OF LABOR

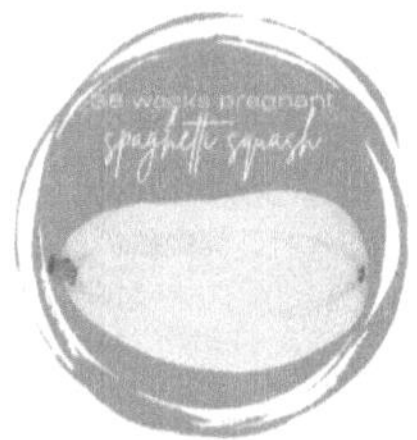

Baby's Size: A spaghetti squash

Mother's Symptoms: Strong Braxton Hicks, increased discharge, lower back pain

What to Expect:

At week 38, your baby is about the size of a spaghetti squash and is continuing to prepare for life outside the womb. They're gaining about half a pound a week and are developing more fat to help regulate their body temperature after birth. Your baby's lungs are fully developed, and they're practicing breathing movements in preparation for their first breath. You might notice that your baby's movements feel different as they have less room to move around.

As your body prepares for labor, you might experience stronger Braxton Hicks contractions that can be confused with real labor contractions. These practice contractions help your body get ready for the real thing. You might also notice an increase in vaginal discharge, which can be a sign that your body is preparing for labor. Lower back pain is common as your baby drops lower into your pelvis, increasing the pressure on your back.

Other Symptoms You Might Experience This Week:

- **Strong Braxton Hicks**: Seeing this in the list must be getting old at this point! You're almost there Momma. These contractions may become more intense and frequent as your body gears up for labor. They're usually irregular and not as intense as real contractions. If they become regular or increase in intensity, it could be a sign that labor is beginning. Time your contractions and contact your healthcare provider if you're unsure.

- **Increased Discharge**: It's normal to experience an increase in vaginal discharge as your body prepares for labor. If you notice a sudden increase or if the discharge is watery, it's important to contact your healthcare provider, as it could indicate that your water has broken.

- **Lower Back Pain**: Lower back pain is common as your baby drops lower into your pelvis. The added pressure can make sitting, standing, and walking uncomfortable. Use a heating pad, practice good posture, and rest as much as possible to alleviate discomfort.

Preparation Tips:

- **Monitor for Signs of Labor**: Be on the lookout for signs of labor, including regular contractions, your water breaking, or lower back pain. If you notice any of these signs, contact your healthcare provider and get ready to head to the hospital or birthing center.

- **Finalize Last-Minute Preparations**: Make sure your hospital bag is packed, the car seat is installed, and your home is ready for your baby's arrival. Double-check that you have all the essentials you'll need for the first few days at home.

- **Stay in Touch with Your Healthcare Provider**: Keep your healthcare provider informed of any changes you notice in your symptoms. They can help guide you through the final days of pregnancy and let you know when it's time to come in.

WEEK 39: READY FOR BABY'S ARRIVAL

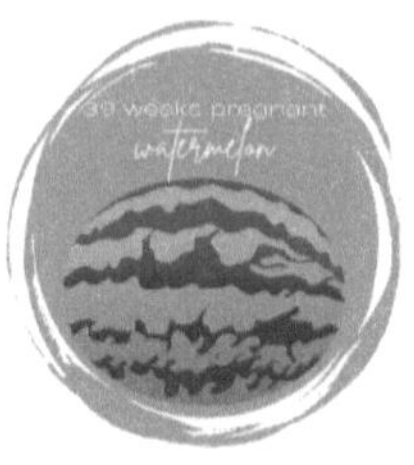

Baby's Size: A watermelon

Mother's Symptoms: Fatigue, **anticipation**, possible water breaking

What to Expect:

At week 39, your baby is about the size of a small watermelon and is fully developed and ready to make their entrance into the world! It could very possibly be go-time at anytime. They're continuing to gain weight, and their skin is becoming smoother as they build up fat stores. Your baby is likely head-down and positioned for birth, with their movements becoming more restricted due to the lack of space.

As your due date approaches, you may feel a mix of emotions—excitement, anticipation, and even a bit of anxiety. Fatigue may return as your body works hard to support both you and your baby during these final days. One of the key signs that labor is imminent is the breaking of your water, which is the rupture of the amniotic sac. If this happens, it's important to contact your healthcare provider immediately, as labor usually follows soon after.

More on the Symptoms You Might Experience This Week:

- **Fatigue**: As you approach your due date, fatigue may return due to the physical demands of late pregnancy. It's important to rest as much as possible and conserve your energy for labor and delivery.
- **Anticipation**: The anticipation of meeting your baby can be overwhelming. Take time to reflect on your pregnancy journey, and try to stay calm and focused as you prepare for labor. Surround yourself with supportive people who can help you through the final days.
- **Possible Water Breaking**: If your water breaks, it's important to contact your healthcare provider right away. This is usually a sign that labor is starting, and you'll need to go to the hospital or birthing center. Your provider will guide you on the next steps, including when to come in.

Preparation Tips:

- **Stay Hydrated and Nourished**: In the final days of pregnancy, it's important to stay hydrated and eat nutrient-rich foods to keep your energy levels up. Focus on small, frequent meals that are easy to digest.

- **Review Your Birth Plan**: Take a final look at your birth plan and discuss it with your healthcare provider. Make sure your support person knows your preferences and is ready to help you during labor.

- **Relax and Rest**: As you wait for labor to begin, take time to relax and rest. Practice deep breathing, meditation, or other relaxation techniques to help you stay calm and focused. Remember that every labor is different, and your healthcare team is there to support you every step of the way.

Personal Story:

Jessica, who was 39 weeks pregnant, shared her experience with anticipation: "The last few days before my due date were a mix of excitement and nerves. I was so ready to meet my baby, but I also felt **so** anxious about the unknowns of labor. I spent a lot of time resting and trying to stay calm. When my water finally broke, it was a rush of emotions—I knew the moment I had been waiting for was finally here. I was so tickled that everything was really happening that I could not stop laughing! Right or wrong, that was the emotion that kept flowing out of me so I laughed all the way to the hospital. The support of my partner and healthcare team made all the difference, and before I knew it, I was holding my baby in my arms."

WEEK 40+: THE BIG DAY IS NEAR!

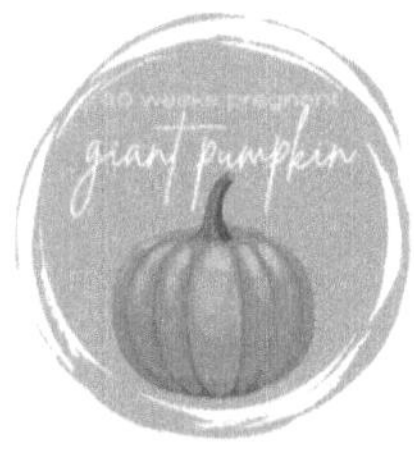

Baby's Size: A big pumpkin

Mother's Symptoms: Fatigue, anticipation, excitement

What to Expect:

You've reached the end of your pregnancy, and your baby is now the size of a big pumpkin! It's been an incredible journey, and you're just days away from meeting your little one. The anticipation is building, and you might be feeling a mix of emotions—fatigue, excitement, and maybe even a bit of anxiety.

If your due date comes and goes without any signs of labor, don't worry—many babies arrive fashionably late. Your healthcare provider will monitor you and your baby closely to ensure everything is going smoothly.

More on the Symptoms You Might Experience This Week:

- **Fatigue**: The final days of pregnancy can be exhausting, both physically and emotionally. Rest as much as you can, and conserve your energy for labor. It's normal to feel a bit anxious as your due date approaches, but try to stay calm and focused on the excitement of meeting your baby.

- **Anticipation**: As you approach your due date, the anticipation can be overwhelming. You've been preparing for this moment for months, and now it's almost here. Take time to reflect on your pregnancy journey and look forward to the incredible experience of bringing your baby into the world.

- **Excitement**: The excitement of knowing that you'll soon be holding your baby in your arms is indescribable. Cherish these final moments of pregnancy, and know that all the discomfort and waiting will be worth it when you finally meet your little one.

Preparation Tips:

- **Discuss induction**: If you go past your due date, talk to your healthcare provider about induction options. They'll help you decide what's best for you and your baby. Induction is usually considered if you're more than a week overdue, but every situation is different.

- **Regular fetal monitoring**: Your provider will likely increase monitoring to ensure your baby is still healthy and active as you wait for labor to begin. This might include non-stress tests or biophysical profiles to check on your baby's well-being.

- **Stay hydrated and rest**: Make sure you're drinking plenty of water and getting as much rest as possible in these final days. Labor is just around the corner, so take care of yourself and get ready for the big moment!

- **Make last-minute home preparations**: Double-check that everything is ready at home for your baby's arrival. This includes having meals prepared, the nursery set up, and your hospital bag by the door. Take some time to relax and enjoy the calm before the excitement of labor and delivery.

Personal Story:

Hannah, who was pregnant with her first child, shared her experience of going past her due date: "I was so sure my baby would arrive on time, but my due date came and went with no sign of labor. It was tough to wait, but my doctor reassured me that everything was fine. I tried to stay busy and distracted, but it was hard not to think about when it would happen. Finally, a week later, I went into labor, and it was such a relief! The waiting was worth it when I finally got to hold my baby."

POSTPARTUM: THE FOURTH TRIMESTER

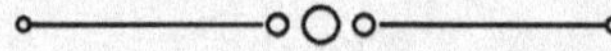

WEEK BY WEEK PREGNANCY GUIDE FOR MODERN MOMS:

HELPFUL FACTS AND EXPERT TIPS FOR EVERY STAGE OF YOUR JOURNEY

By Naomi Knight

WEEKS 1-6: WELCOME TO MOTHERHOOD!

Mother's Recovery: Physical changes, emotional rollercoasters, postpartum care

Baby's Development: Feeding, sleeping (or not!), all the snuggles

What to Expect:

Welcome to the world of motherhood! The first few weeks after your baby arrives are a whirlwind of emotions, physical changes, and incredible moments as you get to know your little one. This is a time that, within a few weeks, will feel like a blur to look back on. If you are into journaling, try to do it in this first month. Your body is recovering from childbirth, and you're learning the ropes of feeding, diapering, and soothing your baby. It's a time of adjustment, but it's also filled with joy, love, and all the snuggles you could ever want.

More on the Symptoms You Might Experience This Week:

- **Physical Recovery**: Your body has just been through an incredible experience, and it needs time to heal. Whether you had a vaginal delivery or a C-section, give yourself grace and time to recover. Rest as much as you can, and don't hesitate to ask for help with household chores or caring for your baby. Use your postpartum care kit to manage discomfort and promote healing.

- **Emotional Rollercoasters**: The postpartum period can be an emotional rollercoaster. Hormonal changes, lack of sleep, and the overwhelming responsibility of caring for a newborn can leave you feeling vulnerable. It's normal to have ups and downs, but if you're feeling persistently sad, anxious, or overwhelmed, talk to your healthcare provider. Postpartum depression is common, and there's help available.

- **Feeding Your Baby**: Whether you're breastfeeding, formula feeding, or a combination of both, feeding your baby is a big part of the postpartum period. Breastfeeding can take some time to get the hang of, so don't hesitate to reach out to a lactation consultant if you need support. If you're formula feeding, follow your baby's cues and feed them on demand. Remember, fed is best, and the most important thing is that your baby is healthy and thriving.

Preparation Tips:

- **Journaling**: I swear your brain's chemistry is adjusting so much, it records very little. Looking back on any photos or videos from the first six weeks of motherhood is surreal, it's like watching someone else! Your memories become so blurry from this incredible time. So try to record as much as possible in the way that you like. Journaling, photos and/or videos will give you all the feels to look through in only a few weeks, and for the rest of your life.

- **Postpartum check-ups**: Make sure to schedule your postpartum check-ups with your healthcare provider. These visits are important for making sure you're healing well and feeling good. Your provider will check your physical recovery, screen for postpartum depression, and answer any questions you have about your new role as a mom.

- **Join a mom group**: Connecting with other new moms can be a lifesaver. Whether it's an in-person group or online, it's great to share tips, experiences, and support during this new chapter. You'll find that you're not alone in your experiences, and the friendships you make can be a source of strength and encouragement.

- **Take care of yourself**: It's easy to focus all your energy on your baby, but don't forget about yourself. Get plenty of rest, eat well, and ask for help when you need it. Make time for self-care, even if it's just a few minutes to relax with a cup of tea or take a short walk. You're doing an amazing job, and taking care of yourself is just as important as taking care of your baby.

Personal Story:

Emily, a mom of two, shared her experience of the postpartum period: "The first few weeks after my baby was born were such a blur. I was exhausted, emotional, and overwhelmed, but I was also completely in love with my baby. What helped me the most was leaning on my support system—my husband, my mom, and my friends. They helped with meals, housework, and even just holding the baby so I could take a shower. It's okay to ask for help, and it's okay to not have everything figured out right away. It gets easier, and every day you learn something new."

APPENDICES

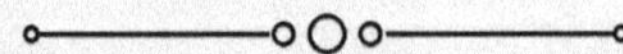

WEEK BY WEEK PREGNANCY GUIDE FOR MODERN MOMS:

HELPFUL FACTS AND EXPERT TIPS FOR EVERY STAGE OF YOUR JOURNEY

By Naomi Knight

GLOSSARY OF PREGNANCY TERMS

Here's a handy glossary of pregnancy terms to help you navigate all the new words and phrases you'll encounter along the way. Knowing the lingo will help you feel more confident and in control throughout your pregnancy.

Amniotic Fluid

The liquid that surrounds and protects the baby in the womb. This fluid helps the baby move around in the uterus, which is important for muscle and bone development.

Braxton Hicks Contractions

These are often called "practice contractions" and can occur throughout pregnancy. Unlike labor contractions, they are irregular and usually don't lead to labor.

Cervix

The lower part of the uterus that opens into the vagina. During pregnancy, it remains closed and thick until labor, when it gradually opens to allow the baby to pass through.

Dilation

The process of the cervix opening during labor, measured in centimeters from 0 to 10. Full dilation (10 cm) is necessary for the baby to pass through the birth canal.

Ectopic Pregnancy

A pregnancy that occurs outside the uterus, usually in a fallopian tube. This type of pregnancy cannot continue to full term and requires medical attention.

Fetal Monitoring

The regular checking of the baby's heart rate, usually during labor, to ensure the baby is healthy and handling the stress of labor well.

Gestational Diabetes

A type of diabetes that develops during pregnancy. It can often be managed with diet and exercise, but sometimes medication is needed.

HCG (Human Chorionic Gonadotropin)

A hormone produced during pregnancy that is detected in pregnancy tests. High levels of HCG are usually an early indicator of pregnancy.

Induction

The process of stimulating labor through medical interventions if labor does not start on its own. This can include medications or other techniques to encourage contractions.

Kick Counts

A way to monitor the baby's activity level by counting the number of movements or kicks felt over a certain period. This can help track the baby's health.

Linea Nigra

A dark line that appears on the belly during pregnancy, running from the belly button to the pubic area. It typically fades after delivery.

Morning Sickness

Nausea and vomiting that many women experience during pregnancy, especially in the first trimester. Despite the name, it can happen at any time of the day.

Nuchal Translucency Scan

An ultrasound test done in the first trimester to measure the thickness of the back of the baby's neck, which can help assess the risk of certain genetic conditions.

Oxytocin

A hormone that plays a role in labor by stimulating contractions and later helps with milk production for breastfeeding.

Placenta

The organ that develops in the uterus during pregnancy, providing oxygen and nutrients to the baby and removing waste products from the baby's blood.

Preterm Labor

Labor that begins before 37 weeks of pregnancy. Babies born preterm may need extra care and time to develop properly.

Quickening

The first movements of the baby that the mother can feel, usually occurring between 16 and 25 weeks of pregnancy.

Round Ligament Pain

Sharp pain or discomfort felt in the lower abdomen or groin area, often during the second trimester. It occurs as the ligaments supporting the uterus stretch and thicken to accommodate the growing baby.

Sonogram (Ultrasound)

An imaging test that uses sound waves to create a picture of the baby inside the womb. It's commonly used to check the baby's development and can sometimes reveal the baby's sex.

Trimester

Pregnancy is divided into three trimesters, each about three months long. Each trimester has its own unique milestones for both the mother and the baby.

Vernix Caseosa

A white, cheesy substance that covers and protects the baby's skin in the womb. It's usually present at birth but is wiped off during the baby's first bath.

Zygote

The fertilized egg that forms after the sperm and egg combine. The zygote then begins to divide and grow into an embryo.

Understanding these terms can help you feel more empowered and prepared as you navigate your pregnancy journey. Remember, knowledge is power, and knowing what's happening at each stage can bring peace of mind as you prepare to welcome your new little one.

SAMPLE BIRTH PLANS

Not sure where to start with your birth plan? Check out these sample birth plans to get ideas and inspiration. Remember, your birth plan is all about what makes you feel comfortable and supported, so make it your own!

Here are three sample birth plans that you can use as inspiration to create your own. Each plan has a different focus based on personal preferences and circumstances.

Sample Birth Plan 1: Minimalist Approach

This birth plan is designed for someone who prefers a straightforward approach with minimal interventions.

Labor Preferences:

- I would like to labor at home as long as possible before going to the hospital.
- Please allow me to move freely and change positions during labor.
- I prefer to use natural pain relief methods such as breathing exercises, walking, and hydrotherapy.

Medical Interventions:

- I would like to avoid an epidural unless I specifically request one.

- Please do not offer pain medications unless I ask for them.
- I prefer to avoid an episiotomy unless absolutely necessary.

Monitoring and Procedures:

- I prefer intermittent fetal monitoring to allow for mobility.
- I would like to avoid an IV unless medically necessary.
- Please delay any unnecessary procedures until after bonding time with my baby.

Delivery Preferences:

- I would like to try different birthing positions, such as squatting or on all fours.
- I prefer a hands-off approach during pushing, allowing my body to do the work.
- I would like my partner to announce the sex of the baby.

Post-Birth Preferences:

- I would like immediate skin-to-skin contact with my baby.
- Please delay cord clamping until the cord has stopped pulsating.

- I would like to breastfeed as soon as possible after birth.

Sample Birth Plan 2: High-Risk Pregnancy

This birth plan is tailored for someone with a high-risk pregnancy who may need more medical interventions but still wants to maintain some control.

Labor Preferences:

- I understand that due to my high-risk status, certain monitoring and interventions may be necessary.
- I prefer to stay mobile as much as possible and would appreciate help with positioning.
- Please discuss any potential interventions with me and my partner before proceeding.

Medical Interventions:

- I am open to an epidural but would like to try managing pain with other methods first.
- If induction becomes necessary, I would prefer to start with less invasive methods, such as membrane stripping or a Foley bulb.

Monitoring and Procedures:

- Continuous fetal monitoring is acceptable, but I would like to avoid being confined to the bed.
- I understand an IV may be necessary, but please keep it as unobtrusive as possible.

Delivery Preferences:

- If a C-section becomes necessary, I would like my partner to be present, and I would appreciate being informed throughout the process.
- If possible, I would like to see and touch my baby immediately after birth, even in the event of a C-section.

Post-Birth Preferences:

- I would like immediate skin-to-skin contact if my baby is healthy.
- If my baby needs to be taken to the NICU, please allow my partner to accompany them.
- I would like to begin breastfeeding as soon as possible, even if it needs to happen in the NICU.

Sample Birth Plan 3: Home Birth with a Midwife

This birth plan is designed for someone planning a home birth with the assistance of a midwife.

Labor Preferences:

- I plan to labor and deliver at home with the support of my midwife and partner.
- I would like to create a calm environment with dim lighting, soft music, and minimal interruptions.
- I prefer to use a birthing pool for pain relief and to assist with delivery.

Medical Interventions:

- I would like to avoid medical interventions unless there is a clear medical need.
- I prefer to avoid any pain medications and would like to use natural methods such as water, massage, and breathing techniques.
- If transfer to a hospital becomes necessary, I would like my midwife to accompany me.

Monitoring and Procedures:

- I prefer intermittent monitoring of the baby's heart rate using a Doppler.
- I would like my midwife to guide me through the pushing stage without excessive coaching.

Delivery Preferences:

- I would like to deliver in a position that feels most comfortable, whether in the birthing pool or another area of the home.
- I prefer for my baby to be placed on my chest immediately after birth without any cleaning or intervention.
- My partner would like to cut the umbilical cord after it has stopped pulsating.

Post-Birth Preferences:

- I would like to delay newborn procedures (e.g., weighing, measuring) until after we have had some time to bond.
- I plan to exclusively breastfeed and would appreciate support with latching if needed.
- I would like to take placenta capsules and would like to keep the placenta after birth.

Remember, your birth plan is personal to you, so feel free to modify these examples to fit your preferences and needs.

You got this momma!

PRENATAL AND POSTNATAL CARE CHECKLIST

This checklist covers all the important prenatal and postnatal care you'll need. From appointments and tests to self-care tips, it's your go-to guide for staying on top of everything during your pregnancy journey.

Prenatal Care Checklist

First Trimester (Weeks 1-12):

- Schedule Initial Prenatal Visit: Meet with your healthcare provider to confirm your pregnancy and discuss your medical history.
- Prenatal Vitamins: Start taking prenatal vitamins with folic acid.
- Initial Blood Work and Tests: Complete routine blood work, including blood type, Rh factor, and screening for infections.
- Healthy Lifestyle: Begin or maintain a healthy diet, regular exercise, and avoid harmful substances like alcohol and tobacco.
- Early Ultrasound: Schedule an ultrasound to confirm your due date and check the baby's development.
- Genetic Screening: Discuss and decide on genetic screening options if desired.

Second Trimester (Weeks 13-27):

- Anatomy Scan: Schedule a mid-pregnancy ultrasound to check your baby's growth and development.
- Glucose Screening Test: Test for gestational diabetes, typically around 24-28 weeks.
- Prenatal Appointments: Continue regular prenatal visits, usually once a month.
- Register for Childbirth Classes: Look into prenatal classes that cover childbirth, breastfeeding, and newborn care.
- Plan for Maternity Leave: Start discussing your maternity leave with your employer.
- Baby Movements: Begin tracking your baby's movements, usually starting around 18-20 weeks.

Third Trimester (Weeks 28-40):

- Group B Strep Test: Get tested for Group B Streptococcus (GBS) around 36 weeks.
- Finalize Birth Plan: Review and finalize your birth plan with your healthcare provider.
- Pack Your Hospital Bag: Include essentials for yourself, your partner, and your baby.
- Prenatal Visits Increase: Attend bi-weekly or weekly prenatal visits as you near your due date.
- Pre-register at Hospital or Birth Center: Ensure your paperwork is complete to avoid any last-minute stress.

- Prepare for Postpartum: Stock up on postpartum supplies and make arrangements for help at home if needed.

Postnatal Care Checklist

Immediately After Birth:

- **Skin-to-Skin Contact**: Spend time bonding with your baby through skin-to-skin contact.
- **First Feeding**: Initiate breastfeeding as soon as possible, with support from the medical team.
- **Newborn Screening Tests**: Ensure your baby undergoes necessary screenings, including hearing and metabolic tests.
- **Postpartum Recovery**: Start using any postpartum care supplies, such as pads or ice packs, to aid your recovery.

First Few Weeks at Home:

- **Newborn Checkup**: Schedule your baby's first pediatrician visit within the first week.
- **Postpartum Checkup**: Make an appointment for your six-week postpartum visit to check on your physical and emotional recovery.
- **Breastfeeding Support**: Reach out to a lactation consultant if you need help with breastfeeding.

- **Rest and Nutrition**: Focus on rest, staying hydrated, and eating nutrient-rich foods to support your recovery.
- **Mental Health Check**: Monitor your emotional well-being and seek support if you experience symptoms of postpartum depression or anxiety.
- **Pelvic Floor Exercises**: Begin gentle pelvic floor exercises when you feel ready, to aid in recovery.

Ongoing Postnatal Care:

- **Vaccinations**: Keep track of your baby's vaccination schedule and attend all necessary appointments.
- **Contraceptive Planning**: Discuss postpartum contraceptive options with your healthcare provider.
- **Postpartum Checkups**: Continue attending any follow-up appointments for both you and your baby.
- **Self-Care**: Make time for activities that promote your physical and mental well-being, such as gentle exercise or relaxation techniques.
- **Social Support**: Stay connected with friends, family, or new parent groups for social support and advice.

This checklist is your go-to guide to ensure you're staying on top of everything during your pregnancy and postpartum journey. Tailor it to your needs, and don't hesitate to ask for help when you need it.

You got this momma.

FINANCIAL PLANNING WORKSHEET FOR NEW PARENTS

Get a head start on planning for your baby's arrival with this financial worksheet. It covers budgeting, expenses, and resources to help you prepare financially for your little one.

This worksheet is designed to help you organize and plan your finances as you prepare for your baby's arrival. It covers key areas like budgeting, tracking expenses, and identifying resources to ensure you're financially ready for this new chapter.

1. Monthly Budget Overview

Income:

Total Monthly Household Income: $ _______

Fixed Monthly Expenses:

Rent/Mortgage: $ _______

Utilities (Electricity, Water, Gas, etc.): $ _______

Insurance (Health, Life, Auto, Home): $ _______

Car Payments: $ _______

Debt Payments (Loans, Credit Cards, etc.): $ _______

Savings Contributions: $ _______

Retirement Contributions: $ _______

Fixed Expenses: $ _______

Total Fixed Monthly Expenses: $

Variable Monthly Expenses:

Groceries: $

Transportation (Gas, Public Transit, etc.): $

Childcare (if applicable): $

Entertainment: $

Dining Out/Takeout: $

Miscellaneous: $

Total Variable Monthly Expenses: $

Total Monthly Expenses (Fixed + Variable): $

**Remaining Monthly Income
(Income - Total Expenses):** $

2. Baby-Related Expenses

One-Time Baby Expenses:

Nursery Setup (Crib, Changing Table, etc.): $

Car Seat: $

Stroller: $

Baby Clothes: $

Baby Gear (High Chair, Carrier, etc.): $

Diapering Supplies (Cloth/Disposable): $

Feeding Supplies (Bottles, Breast Pump, etc.): $

Maternity Wardrobe: $

Hospital/Midwife Fees: $ _______

Total One-Time Baby Expenses: $ _______

Ongoing Baby Expenses:

Diapers (Monthly): $ _______

Baby Formula/Breastfeeding Supplies (Monthly): $ _______

Baby Food (Starting after 6 months): $ _______

Childcare (Monthly, if applicable): $ _______

Medical Expenses (Pediatrician visits, etc.): $ _______

Clothing & Toys (Monthly): $ _______

Total Ongoing Monthly Baby Expenses: $ _______

3. Emergency Fund Planning

Current Emergency Fund Balance: $ _______

Emergency Fund Goal

(3-6 months of living expenses): $ _______

Additional Contributions Needed to Reach Goal: $ _______

Monthly Contribution Amount: $ _______

4. Insurance Review

Health Insurance:

Current Coverage (Individual/Family Plan): $ _______

Monthly Premium: $ _______

Out-of-Pocket Costs (Deductibles, Copays, etc.): $ _______

Life Insurance:

Current Policy Coverage: $

Monthly Premium: $

Disability Insurance:

Current Policy Coverage: $

Monthly Premium: $

Review Notes:

5. Income Adjustments & Parental Leave

Maternity/Paternity Leave:

Planned Start Date:

Duration of Leave:

Income During Leave: $

Adjustments to Income:

Short-Term Disability Payments (if applicable): $

Employer-Provided Benefits (if applicable): $

Other Sources of Income: $

6. Long-Term Financial Planning

College Savings:

Current College Savings Balance: $

Monthly Contribution Goal: $ _______

College Savings Plan (e.g., 529): _______________________

Retirement Savings:

Current Retirement Savings Balance: $ _______

Monthly Contribution Goal: $ _______

7. Financial Resources & Support

Government Assistance (if applicable):

WIC (Women, Infants, and Children): $ _______

SNAP (Supplemental Nutrition

Assistance Program): $ _______

Medicaid: $ _______

Community Resources:

Local Parenting Groups: $ _______

Free/Discounted Baby Supplies: $ _______

Other Financial Support:

Family Contributions: $ _______

Grants/Scholarships: $ _______

8. Notes & Action Items

This worksheet is your financial roadmap as you prepare for parenthood. Use it to track your expenses, set savings goals, and ensure you're ready for the financial responsibilities that come with welcoming your little one.

RESOURCES AND FURTHER READING

Looking for more information? Check out this curated list of books, websites, and other resources to guide you through every step of your pregnancy and parenting journey. Whether you're planning, expecting, or navigating life with a newborn, these resources are here to help!

Books:

"First Time Pregnancy for Modern Moms: From Planning to Delivery" by Naomi Knight (hey that's me!)

A The most up-to-date expert information for a joyful and stress-free first pregnancy. How to find the right kind of care for yourself and how to make important decisions that will come up during pregnancy and birth.

"The Happiest Baby on the Block" by Dr. Harvey Karp

Discover techniques for soothing your baby and getting more sleep during those challenging early months.

"Bringing Up Bébé" by Pamela Druckerman

An insightful look at French parenting techniques, focusing on raising well-behaved, self-sufficient children.

"Ina May's Guide to Childbirth" by Ina May Gaskin

A must-read for those interested in natural birth, filled with empowering birth stories and expert advice.

"The Baby Book" by Dr. William Sears and Martha Sears

A go-to resource on attachment parenting, offering guidance on breastfeeding, sleep, and babywearing.

"Cribsheet" by Emily Oster

A data-driven approach to parenting, breaking down the research behind common parenting decisions.

Websites:

[BabyCenter](https://www.babycenter.com)

Offers a wealth of articles, forums, and tools to track your pregnancy and baby's development.

[The Bump](https://www.thebump.com)

A great resource for week-by-week pregnancy advice, baby gear reviews, and parenting tips.

[La Leche League International](https://www.llli.org)

Provides support and information for breastfeeding moms, including local groups and online forums.

[KellyMom](https://www.kellymom.com)

Evidence-based breastfeeding and parenting information written by an experienced lactation consultant.

[HealthyChildren.org](https://www.healthychildren.org)
    Run by the American Academy of Pediatrics, this site
    offers expert advice on child health and safety.

[Spinning Babies](https://www.spinningbabies.com)
    Focuses on optimal fetal positioning and techniques
    for a smoother, more comfortable birth experience.

Apps:

Pregnancy Tracker - BabyCenter - Ovia
    Track your baby's development week by week and get
    tips for each stage of pregnancy.

The Wonder Weeks
    Understand your baby's mental development and track
    their progress through key developmental milestones.

Peanut
    Connect with other moms and moms-to-be in your
    area, ask questions, and share experiences.

Glow Nurture
    A personalized pregnancy tracker with daily health
    insights, checklists, and community support.

Baby Connect
    An all-in-one app to track your baby's feedings, sleep,
    and milestones, perfect for staying organized during
    those busy first months.

Podcasts:

"The Birth Hour"
Listen to real birth stories from moms around the world, offering inspiration and insights into different birthing experiences.

"The Longest Shortest Time"
A podcast about the surprises, joys, and challenges of parenting, with stories from all walks of life.

"Pregnancy Podcast"
Weekly episodes that explore all aspects of pregnancy, childbirth, and postpartum, with evidence-based information.

"Happy as a Mother"
Focuses on maternal mental health, offering advice and support for new moms.

"The Double Shift"
Explores the culture of motherhood, work-life balance, and the experiences of working moms.

Support Groups:

La Leche League

Join a local chapter or online group to get breastfeeding support and connect with other nursing moms.

Postpartum Support International (PSI)

Provides resources and support for postpartum mental health, including online support groups and a helpline.

Babywearing International

Connect with local babywearing groups to learn about safe and effective babywearing techniques.

MOPS (Mothers of Preschoolers)

A community for moms with young children, offering meetups, support, and resources for navigating early motherhood.

CONCLUSION:
YOUR INCREDIBLE JOURNEY INTO PARENTHOOD

Family Planning and Pregnancy can be such a long road. You've come so far, and now you're about to begin the most amazing adventure of all—parenthood! It's been a wild ride, full of ups and downs, but every moment has brought you closer to meeting your beautiful baby.

As you step into this new chapter, remember that **you've got this, momma.** Trust yourself, lean on your support system, and enjoy every moment of this incredible journey. Parenthood is full of surprises, but it's also full of joy, love, and unforgettable memories. You're going to be a phenomenal parent, and your baby is so lucky to have you!

Congratulations 🎉 and welcome to the wonderful world of parenthood!

THANK YOU

Hey, gorgeous momma, I just want to say a heartfelt thank you for reading my book!

Free or paid, there are a LOT of books out there on pregnancy and parenting that I know you could have chosen, and I'm grateful you picked my book for your journey.

So thanks - not only for getting this book but for *finishing* it!

I would be so appreciative if you'll consider posting a review on the platform. The best and easiest way to support the work of independent authors like myself is by leaving a review.

I want to keep writing the kind of books that will help you get the information you want, and your feedback will help me on this path. It would mean so much to me to see your comment under this book!

Thanks and all my best to you, momma-to-be 🤍
Naomi

>> <u>**Leave a review on Amazon US**</u> <<
>> <u>**Leave a review on Amazon UK**</u> <<